Study Design and Statistical Analysis
A Practical Guide for Clinicians

This book takes the reader through the entire res... designing a study, collecting the data, using univa... ...s, and publishing the results. It does so by using plain language rather than complex derivations and mathematical formulae. It focuses on the nuts and bolts of performing research by asking and answering the most basic questions about doing research studies. It has numerous tables, graphs and tips to help demystify the process. It is filled with up-to-date examples from the clinical literature on how to use statistical analyses to answer important questions.

Study Design and Statistical Analysis

A Practical Guide for Clinicians

Mitchell H. Katz

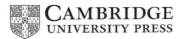

CAMBRIDGE
UNIVERSITY PRESS

CAMBRIDGE UNIVERSITY PRESS
Cambridge, New York, Melbourne, Madrid, Cape Town, Singapore, São Paulo, Delhi

Cambridge University Press
The Edinburgh Building, Cambridge CB2 8RU, UK

Published in the United States of America by Cambridge University Press, New York

www.cambridge.org
Information on this title: www.cambridge.org/9780521826756

©M.H. Katz 2006

First published 2006
Reprinted 2009

Printed in the United Kingdom at the University Press, Cambridge

A catalog record for this publication is available from the British Library

Library of Congress Cataloging in Publication data

ISBN 978-0-521-82675-4 hardback
ISBN 978-0-521-53407-9 paperback

To best friends: Perri Klass and Adam Lowe

Contents

Preface

I decided to write this book based on the many favorable responses I received about my first book: *Multivariable Analysis: A Practical Guide for Clinicians.* Readers who found the conceptual, non-mathematical approach to multivariable analysis helpful, asked me to write a basic statistics book using the same format. My hope is that the two books together will enable clinical researchers to design rigorous studies and analyse the data using both basic and advanced statistical techniques. Although oriented for researchers performing their own studies, the book will also enable readers of clinical research to understand how statistics are used – and misused – in the published literature.

My experience teaching statistics has led me to believe that most statistics textbooks present the material backwards. Typically the formulas and derivations are presented first; only after you have slogged your way through the mathematics are you rewarded with the fun part – analyzing data to answer important questions. The problem with this approach is that many readers will be bored or overwhelmed during the mathematical approach, and will have lost interest in the subject before they get to the fun part.

I have tried to do the opposite by putting the fun part first. I have included clinical examples at the beginning and throughout the text so that you can experience the intellectual pleasure of identifying a question and using statistical analyses to answer it. To ensure that the book would not be intimidating I have excluded derivations, minimized the use of algebraic expressions, and, where possible, used words rather than mathematical symbols to express the underlying statistical concepts. As readily available statistical programs, such as Stata or SAS or Epi Info, will correctly perform the mathematics for you, I think that what is most important is to understand the concepts.

Once hooked on clinical research I hope you will want to learn more. An excellent book that includes derivations and a more thorough review of many of the concepts discussed in this book is: S. Glantz's *Primer of Biostatistics* (5th edition, McGraw-Hill, 2001). For a more comprehensive approach, I recommend B. Rosner's *Fundamentals of Biostatistics* (5th edition, Duxbury, 2000).

I have organized the book to fit the chronologic order of how clinical research is performed: identification of a question, study design, data collection, univariate, bivariate, and multivariable analysis, manuscript writing and publication of the results. This organization should allow you to read each chapter as you are working on that part of the study.

One exception to the chronologic order of this book is that I have placed the sample size section after the section on statistics. Even though you will need to determine the needed sample size prior to collecting and analyzing your data, you can't calculate a sample size without knowing what type of statistical analysis you will be performing.

As much as possible I have included practical advice on the nuts and bolts of performing clinical research, such as how to recode and transform variables. This information is rarely included in statistics books but if done incorrectly will lead you to the wrong answer.

I have minimized overlap between this book and my multivariable book, just released in a new 2nd edition (Cambridge University Press, 2005). If you want to know more about multivariable analysis than contained in Chapter 6, I hope you will read it.

In writing this book I am indebted to my teachers, students, and colleagues. I include among my teachers several epidemiologists and biostatisticians I have never met but whose books I have benefited from. Rather than name them all here I have cited them liberally in the footnotes. One reference I found particularly helpful at several points was B.S. Everett's *Medical Statistics from A to Z* (Cambridge University Press, 2003). My colleagues at the Department of Public Health and the University of San Francisco, California have taught me much about identifying and answering important clinical questions. Several years of students in the University of California, San Francisco, Training in Clinical Research Program have sharpened my teaching skills by letting me try out different methods of presenting the material. Warren Browner, Susan Buchbinder, Jeffrey Martin, and Rani Marx reviewed the manuscript and made many helpful suggestions. If any errors crept in despite their review, I alone am to blame.

In writing this book, I appreciate the support of my editor Peter Silver and the staff at Cambridge University Press.

If you have questions of suggestions for future editions e-mail me at mhkatz59@yahoo.com

1

Introduction

1.1 Why is statistical analysis so important for clinical research?

Most treatments are not sufficiently effective for you to tell whether or not they work based solely on clinical experience. You need statistical analysis!

Consider the question of whether or not to anticoagulate patients with atrial fibrillation (a condition where the heart beats irregularly) and normal heart valves. Such patients are predisposed to emboli (blood clots that travel to other parts of the body). Although anticoagulation with warfarin prevents strokes due to emboli, it can cause serious side effects (bleeding). So what do you do if you have a patient with atrial fibrillation and normal heart valves?

I remember distinctly how Dr. Kanu Chatterjee, one of the greatest cardiologists to have ever practiced medicine, answered this question in 1987. I was among the medical residents congregated around him at University of California, San Francisco Medical Center waiting for pearls of wisdom. He took a deep breath and said: "What you do is you anticoagulate all your patients with atrial fibrillation until one of them bleeds into his head. Then you don't anticoagulate any of your patients until one of them has a stroke. Then you go back to anticoagulating all of them."

Dr. Chatterjee was admitting with an honesty and humility often missing in clinical medicine that it was not clear whether the benefits of anticoagulation outweighed the risks. He was also capturing the tendency of physicians to base their decisions, in the absence of definitive evidence, on their most recent experience.

Fifteen years later, a pooled analysis of six randomized clinical trials demonstrated that anticoagulation with warfarin was superior to aspirin for patients with atrial fibrillation and normal heart valves (Table 1.1).[1]

Note that the risk of ischemic stroke is lower with warfarin (2.0 events per 100 patient-years) than with aspirin (4.3 events per 100 patient-years). Although the

---

[1] van Walraven, C., Hart, R.G., Singer, D.E., et al. Oral anticoagulants versus aspirin in nonvalvular atrial fibrillation: an individual patient meta-analysis. *J. Am. Med. Assoc.* 2002; 288: 2441–8.

Table 1.1. Should you anticoagulate persons with atrial fibrillation and normal heart values?

	Events per 100 patient-years	
	Warfarin	Aspirin
Rate of ischemic stroke	2.0	4.3
Rate of major bleed	2.2	1.3

Data from van Walraven, C., et al. Oral anticoagulants versus aspirin in nonvalvular atrial fibrillation: an individual patient meta-analysis. *J. Am. Med. Assoc.* 2002; 228: 2441–8.

> Statistics are needed to quantify differences that are too small to recognize through clinical experience alone.

risk of a major bleed is higher with warfarin (2.2 events per 100 patient-years) than with aspirin (1.3 events per 100 patient-years) this increase is smaller than the decrease in ischemic strokes. No cardiologist, no matter how many patients with atrial fibrillation he or she has cared for and no matter how careful he or she is at tracking the outcomes of those patients, could recognize such small but important differences through experience alone.

Even if you had the ability to detect such small differences in clinical outcomes you would still need statistics to determine whether the detected difference was greater than the difference you would expect by chance. After all, you would not expect the experience of patients receiving anticoagulation to be exactly the same as those not receiving anticoagulation. There would be some difference. The important question is whether the difference reflects a true difference between the two groups or random (chance) variation.

To understand how statistical analysis helps us evaluate the role of chance in producing differences between groups, let us consider a familiar example: the flip of a coin.

If you flip a coin that is equally weighted on both sides a hundred times (sample size, also known as N, of 100) it will land on heads *about* 50 times and tails *about* 50 times. I have italicized "about" because it represents chance intruding on truth. The truth is that an equally weighted coin should produce an equal number of heads and tails. But because of chance you may not get an equal number of heads and tails. Instead you may get 51 heads and 49 tails, or 49 heads and 51 tails, or 48 heads and 52 tails, etc. None of these results would make you suspicious that the coin was more heavily weighted on one side than the other.

But if the coin lands too often on a particular side, you will get suspicious as to whether the coin really is equally weighted. At a certain point, you will conclude that the difference between the results you were expecting (50–50) and the results that the coin is producing are so great that it cannot be due to chance.

Table 1.2. What result with 100 tosses would make you believe that the coin is not equally weighted on both sides?

100 tosses		
Heads, N (%)	Tails, N (%)	Probability*
50 (50)	50 (50)	1.0
49 (49)	51 (51)	0.92
48 (48)	52 (52)	0.69
45 (45)	55 (55)	0.32
40 (40)	60 (60)	0.05
35 (35)	65 (65)	0.003

* Probability of the observed data (or a more extreme result in either direction) when the expected probability for heads/tails is 0.50.

Table 1.2 quantifies what you already know intuitively. It shows the probability of obtaining a variety of results (or a more extreme result) assuming that an equally weighted coin is flipped 100 times.

You can see that with 100 tosses even a distribution as unequal as 45% heads and 55% tails has a good chance of being due to chance alone (0.32 or about 1 in 3 trials). This probability is too high to conclude confidently that the coin is weighted more heavily on one side. However, if you have a more disproportionate distribution of 40% heads and 60% tails the probability that the result is due to chance is markedly smaller (0.05 or about 1 in 20 trials). By convention, a probability (*P*-value) of less than 0.05 is said to be *statistically significant*. In other words, unlikely to be due to chance. Whether you use the conventional cut-off of $P < 0.05$ or a more or less stringent one depends in part on the harm that would come from being wrong (i.e., rejecting the null hypothesis when it is correct or accepting the null hypothesis when it is wrong).

You will find that when sample sizes are large, even small differences are statistically significant. For example, the probability of obtaining a particular result (or a more extreme one) if you flip a coin 1000 times is shown in Table 1.3. Note, that with 1000 flips, having 45% land on heads results in a low probability ($P = 0.002$) that chance is the correct explanation of the results. Compare this to Table 1.2. When we had only 100 flips we could not reject the null hypothesis with a split of 45% and 55%. This should not surprise you. With more flips (a larger sample size) you have more data on which to make a determination that the coin is not acting as you would expect it to. Therefore, with larger sample sizes smaller differences from what would be expected will tip you off that the coin is not equally weighted.

> By convention, a probability (*P*-value) of less than 0.05 is said to be *statistically significant*.

Table 1.3. What result with 1000 tosses would make you believe that the coin is not weighted equally on both sides?

1000 tosses		
Heads, N (%)	Tails, N (%)	Probability*
500 (50)	500 (50)	1.0
490 (49)	510 (51)	0.52
480 (48)	520 (52)	0.22
450 (45)	550 (55)	0.002
400 (40)	600 (60)	<0.001
350 (35)	650 (65)	<0.001

* Refer to footnote of Table 1.2.

Table 1.4. What result with ten tosses would make you believe that the coin is not weighted equally on both sides?

10 tosses		
Heads, N (%)	Tails, N (%)	Probability*
5 (50)	5 (50)	1.0
4 (40)	6 (60)	0.75
2 (20)	8 (80)	0.11
1 (10)	9 (90)	0.02
0 (0)	10 (100)	0.002

* Refer to footnote of Table 1.2.

Conversely, with small samples even large differences could occur by chance alone. For example, if you toss a coin only 10 times a 20%/80% split could occur with an equally weighted coin due to chance alone with a reasonably high frequency ($P = 0.11$ or 1 in 9 times) (Table 1.4). It is only when you reach a 10%/90% split that the probability dips below the conventional threshold for rejecting the null hypothesis ($P < 0.05$).

The coin toss example illustrates that the two key elements in determining whether a result is due to chance are (1) the magnitude of the difference from what would be expected by chance; and (2) the sample size.

The more a result differs from what would be expected by chance and the larger the sample size, the more likely it is that the result cannot be explained by chance. When a result is unlikely to be due to chance you can consider alternative

> The two key elements in determining whether a result is due to chance are the magnitude of the difference from what would be expected by chance and the size of the sample.

explanations. In the case of the coin toss example, if the probability of a particular result is very low, you can consider the possibility that you are dealing with an unfair coin.

A similar process occurs when considering whether two variables are associated with one another. For example, Ponsky and colleagues assessed whether health insurance status was associated with appendiceal rupture in children.[2] Appendiceal rupture occurs when an infected appendix is not removed quickly enough. Children without private health insurance may not be taken to the doctor when they have the early mild symptoms of appendicitis because they have poor access to care.

To assess an association between two variables, we begin by assuming that the null hypothesis is true. The null hypothesis is that there is no association between two variables, or no difference between two or more groups. In this case, the null hypothesis is that there is no association between having private health insurance and appendiceal rupture in children.

Having stated the null hypothesis we collect data to see if we can reject the null hypothesis. The ability to reject the null hypothesis when it is false is referred to as the power of a study.

Ponsky and colleagues used administrative data from 36 pediatric hospitals in the USA to assess the association between having private health insurance and appendiceal rupture. They found that appendiceal rupture was less likely to occur among privately insured children (32%) than children without private insurance (44%) (Table 1.5). But is it possible that the association between insurance status and appendiceal rupture is solely due to chance sampling of the underlying population? After all, this sample of 18,312 children is just one of an infinite number of samples that could be taken of children with appendicitis.

Although each such sample would likely produce a (slightly or very) different association between insurance status and appendiceal rupture, the question we need to answer is: how likely is it that we could get the data seen in Table 1.5, if there were no true association between health insurance status and appendiceal rupture?

To answer this question we perform a chi-squared analysis (Section 5.2). The small P-value of the chi-squared tells you that it is very unlikely that we would have gotten a sample with the data shown in Table 1.5, if there were no association between insurance status and appendiceal rupture in the population.

> **Definition**
>
> The null hypothesis is that there is no association between two variables, or no difference between two or more groups.

> **Definition**
>
> Power is the ability to reject the null hypothesis when it is false.

---

[2] Ponsky, T.A., Huang, Z.J., Kittle, K., et al. Hospital- and patient-level characteristics and the risk of appendiceal rupture and negative appendectomy in children. *J. Am. Med. Assoc.* 2004; 292: 1977–82.

Table 1.5. Association of insurance status with appendiceal rupture in children

	Appendiceal rupture	
Private health insurance	Yes	No
Yes	3085 (32)	6644 (68)
No	3804 (44)	4779 (56)

Chi-squared *P*-value = 0.002.

Values represented as *N* (%).

Data from Ponsky, T.A., Huang, Z.J., Kittle, K., et al. Hospital-
and patient-level characteristics and the risk of appendiceal rupture and
negative appendectomy in children. *J. Am. Med. Assoc.* 2004; 292: 1977–82.

Definition

Inferential statistics are used to draw conclusions about populations from samples of those populations.

Statistics (such as the chi-squared) that are used to draw conclusions about populations from samples are referred to as inferential statistics. We infer the truth about the population from the findings in the sample.

Having eliminated chance sampling from the population as the reason for this association, we can consider the alternative explanation: that there is an association between insurance status and appendiceal rupture.

A common mistake at this point in the process is to assume that if there is an association, the association is causal (i.e., not having health insurance leads to delays in appendectomy). But causality is only one alternative explanation of an association that is not due to chance. Another alternative explanation is confounding (i.e., the apparent association between two variables is actually due to a third variable or variables, Section 2.3.A). In the case of this study, there is a possibility that low income, which is associated with insurance status, may be the true cause of the higher rate of appendiceal rupture. Another alternative explanation is reverse causality (i.e., the "effect" causes the "cause", Section 2.6.A). This is an unlikely explanation in this case, since it is hard to imagine how having appendiceal rupture would lead to not having private insurance, but reverse causality may be true in other instances. Finally, bias (systematic error in measurement due to flaws in the design and/or conduct of the study, Section 2.3.B) is an issue in all studies. For example, bias could affect the results if uninsured children with appendiceal rupture were more likely to be transferred to one of the hospitals in this sample than insured children with appendiceal rupture.

The best way to eliminate these other alternative explanations is through rigorous study design. Therefore, I have placed the chapter on study design (Chapter 2), ahead of the chapters on statistical analysis. Other strategies for strengthening causal inference are discussed in Section 9.2.

Another common mistake is to assume that your results can be generalized to (can be assumed to be true for) other populations than the one that was sampled (Section 2.4). For example, Ponsky and colleagues drew their sample from the population of children having appendectomies. Whether adults without health insurance are also more likely to have appendiceal rupture than insured adults cannot be answered by their data. (But has been answered in the affirmative by other studies![3])

---

[3] Braveman, P., Schaaf, V.M., Egerter, S., Bennett, T., Schecter, W. Insurance-related differences in the risk of ruptured appendix. *New Engl. J. Med.* 1994; 331: 444–9.

2 Designing a study

2.1 How do I choose a research question?

The first step in designing a study is to formulate a research question. Most clinical researchers appropriately wish to study a question in their field of practice. But knowing that you want to do a research project in a field such as HIV/AIDS or cardiology or orthopedics, is quite different than having a research question. For example: What about HIV/AIDS, are you interested in studying? Methods of preventing infection? How to diagnose infection? The prevalence of infection? Survival with HIV/AIDS? The frequency of specific HIV/AIDS manifestations?

One of the best ways to identify a research question is to determine what the unknowns are in your field. What do you and the other clinicians in your field wish you knew but don't? Perhaps your clinical experience suggests to you that a particular condition is more common in one population than another, but you're not sure if your clinical experience is typical or not. Perhaps you've evaluated a patient with a particular symptom and found that the literature lacked compelling data on how to treat the patient or what test to perform next.

Research questions may be descriptive or analytic. As implied by the name, descriptive questions focus on explaining clinical phenomena such as prevalence of disease (e.g., What is the prevalence of HIV among homeless persons?), survival trends (e.g., What is the proportion of men with prostate cancer who are alive at 5 years?), health service utilization (What is the proportion of seniors receiving influenza (flu) vaccination?), and clinical test characteristics (e.g., What is the mean value of D-dimer levels among patients who have had a venous thromboembolism?).

Analytic questions are comparative: For example: Is HIV prevalence higher among homeless persons than among housed persons? Is survival among men with prostate cancer better with surgery or radiation? Are seniors with health insurance more likely to receive flu vaccine than uninsured seniors? Are persons with higher D-dimer levels more likely to have a recurrent venous thromboembolism than patients with lower levels?

In general, analytic questions are more interesting than descriptive ones because answering them may enable us to develop interventions to prevent disease or better target interventions to particular populations. However, descriptive questions often must be answered first. For example, without a thorough understanding of the baseline frequency of a condition, it may be impossible to design a study to answer an analytic question.

Whether you are answering a descriptive or analytic question, specify the population in which you will be answering the question: men, women, elders, youth, homeless persons, etc.

In choosing a research question, remember that life is short and the time it takes to complete research projects is long. (The median time between the start of enrollment of subjects and the publication of results was found to be 5.5 years for randomized controlled efficacy trials.[4]) Choose a question for which your excitement is sufficient to sustain you through tedious protocol revisions, temperamental collaborators, protective human subjects review committees, lagging enrollment, subjects who drop out of your study, missing data, writer's block, slow journal editors, jealous reviewers, and the myriad of other obstacles to performing and publishing good research.

Try to choose a research question that will have an impact on the health and well being of a population you care about. Sometimes researchers get so caught up in the academic game of grantsmanship, publication, and promotion, that they lose sight that the purpose of clinical research is to improve health by identifying risk factors of disease, improving diagnoses, finding new treatments, etc. Much well-done health care research is published that has no impact on health care.

A turning point in my research career was a study I performed on temporal trends in AIDS-related opportunistic infections.[5] At the time, clinicians noted a change in the pattern of opportunistic infections and malignancies in patients with AIDS. Specifically, with the advent of prophylaxis for *Pneumocystis carinii* pneumonia, the rate of other opportunistic infections for which we had no form of prophylaxis at that time, such as disseminated *Mycobacterium avium* complex and cytomegalovirus were increasing. I used data from a natural history cohort to determine the rate of the different manifestations by calendar year.

From an academic point of view, the study was a success. It got accepted for publication on the first submission to the leading infectious disease journal. I had

---

[4] Ioannidis, J.P. Effect of the statistical significance of results on the time to completion and publication of randomized efficacy trials. *J. Am. Med. Assoc.* 1998; 279: 281–6.
[5] Katz, M.H., Hessol, N.A., Buchbinder, S.P., et al. Temporal trends of opportunistic infections and malignancies in homosexual men with AIDS. *J. Infect. Dis.* 1994; 170: 198–202.

reason to feel pleased with myself, but I wasn't. By the time the paper appeared in print, I realized it made no discernable difference in the care of persons with HIV/AIDS. All I had done was to quantitate the rate at which people were developing (then) unpreventable infections. I vowed to myself that I would focus my future research efforts on research that was more likely to have an impact.

Of course, it is sometimes difficult to fully appreciate the impact a study will have before you do it. Also, there have been instances when a study that had no immediate impact turned out to be influential in moving a field forward many years later. Nonetheless, the chance that your work will have an impact is greater if you address an important clinical question.

Another way to ensure that the results of your study will matter is to enroll a sufficient number of subjects (Chapter 7) so that a null result is meaningful. A study that detects no difference between two groups, but does not have a sufficient sample size to rule out a meaningful difference, is of no use.

In choosing a research question, consider what questions you are in a particularly good position to answer based on the prevalence of the disease in your area, your prior experience, your colleagues, and your community contacts. It is not a coincidence that most of the research on Burkett's lymphoma is performed in Africa or that most of the research on esophageal cancer is performed in Japan.

Finally, before devoting too much time to your research question, be sure it has not already been answered. This has become significantly easier in the age of computerized literature searches. Pub Med (http://www.ncbi.nlm.nih.gov/PubMed/) is a great resource. It places the holdings of the National Library of Medicine at your fingertips, free of charge.

It is also worth consulting with others in the field to see if a similar study is underway or has been presented at a conference (unfortunately not all abstracts and/or proceedings are electronically accessible).

Although, it is rare that a single study definitively answers a question, it is much less exciting to perform a study that has already been done, unless you are sure you can do it better!

In summary, before undertaking a research project, ask yourself:

Am I truly interested in knowing the results?

Will the results have an impact on clinical practice?

Will I have enough study subjects to answer the question?

Am I in a particularly good position to answer the question?

Has this question already been answered sufficiently well?

If your answers are Yes, Yes, Yes, Yes, and No, get to work choosing a study design![6]

---

[6] For more on choosing a research question, see Hulley, S.B., Cummings, S.R., Browner, W.S., Grady, D., Hearst, N., Newman, T.B. *Designing Clinical Research* (2nd edition). Philadelphia: Lippincott Williams & Wilkins, 2001, pp. 17–24.

Table 2.1. Which study design generally has the greater advantage?

	Randomized study	Observational study
Eliminating confounding	X	
Minimizing bias	X	
Increasing generalizability		X
Speed in conducting study		X
Minimizing expense		X
Addressing a broader range of questions		X

2.2 How do I choose a study design?

There is no one best study design. You need to determine the best study design to answer your question keeping in mind that "best" must take into account feasibility, cost, length of time it will take to complete the study, and the risks and benefits to study participants. Ultimately, most clinical questions are resolved based on multiple studies using a variety of different methodologies.

Distinguishing the different study designs is complicated by the fact that different authors use different classifications and terms to describe the available study designs. I find it easiest to divide studies into randomized versus observational studies (Section 2.3), and then distinguish the different types within these two broad categories (Sections 2.4–2.6).

2.3 What are the differences between randomized and observational studies?

In a randomized design, the investigator manipulates the condition or group assignment. Subjects may be randomized to two or more groups. Typically, one group receives a treatment and the other group receives a different treatment or a placebo. In an observational study the investigator assesses a population without altering the condition or group assignment of the participants.

Randomized and observational studies have different advantages and disadvantages. Randomized studies are generally better at dealing with confounding and bias but have less generalizability, are slower to conduct and more expensive, and cannot answer as broad a range of questions as observational studies (Table 2.1).

2.3.A Eliminating confounding

Confounding occurs when the apparent association between a risk factor and an outcome is affected by the relationship of a third variable to the risk factor

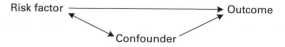

Figure 2.1   Relationship among risk factor, confounder, and outcome.

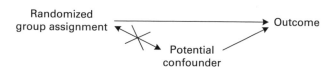

Figure 2.2   With randomization there should be no relationship between confounder and
                             group assignment.

> **Definition**
>
> A confounder is
> associated with the risk
> factor and is causally
> related to the outcome.

and to the outcome; the third variable is called a confounder. For a variable to
be a confounder, the variable must be associated with the risk factor and
causally related to the outcome (Figure 2.1).

For example, several observational studies have shown that elderly persons
who participate in challenging cognitive activities are less likely to develop
dementia. Based solely on this evidence, can you advise your patients that if they
play bridge and do crossword puzzles they are less likely to become demented?
No. The reason is that there are many potential confounders. For example, persons with higher educational attainment and/or cognitive function at baseline
may be more likely to engage in mentally challenging activities. Also persons
with higher education and greater cognitive function may be less likely to
develop dementia because they are starting out at a higher level.

To minimize confounding due to education and cognition you could use
multivariable analysis (Chapter 6). For example, Verghese and colleagues found
that community dwelling elders who engaged in cognitively-demanding leisure
activities were less likely to develop dementia than elders who did not engage in
such activities after statistical adjustment for baseline educational level and cognitive function.[7] Still as the authors acknowledge, there is a possibility that some
other variable confounded their results.

To minimize the possibility that confounding muddies your results, you need
to randomize subjects. To see why compare Figure 2.2 to Figure 2.1. I have put
an X through the line between randomized group assignment and potential
confounder because if your randomization is done correctly there will be no

---

[7] Verghese, J., Lipton, R.B., Katz, M.J., et al. Leisure activities and the risk of dementia in the elderly.
New Engl. J. Med. 2003; 348: 2508–16.

Table 2.2. Strategies for limiting bias in randomized trials

Bias	Strategies for limiting
Steering certain patients into particular treatment groups	Group assignments should be made by a coordinating center with no contact with subjects
Expectations of investigators	Blind investigators to treatment assignment
Expectations of subjects	Blind subjects to treatment assignment Placebos that look and taste the same as the treatment

Randomization eliminates confounding due to known and unknown confounders.

relationship between the two. As long as the randomization is unbiased, your randomized groups will be equal with respect to confounders. Note also that randomization will eliminate confounding whether it is due to a known or an unknown (a measured or unmeasured) confounder. It doesn't matter. The ability to adjust for both known and unknown confounders is a great advantage of randomization because other techniques for minimizing confounding (matching, stratification, multivariable adjustment) can only help with known confounders.

To demonstrate that the relationship between performing cognitive activities and being less likely to develop dementia is not due to confounding, Ball and colleagues randomized elderly persons to cognitive training versus a control group.[8] Participants randomized to cognitive training (memory and reasoning training) showed higher cognitive function 2 years after randomization than those randomized to the control group.

2.3.B Minimizing bias

Definition

Bias is systematic error.

Bias (systematic error) is an issue in both randomized and observational studies and can occur at all stages of a study (e.g., selection of subjects, measurements of subjects, follow-up of subjects).

However, with randomized studies there are several techniques we can use to minimize bias that are not generally applicable to observational studies (Table 2.2).

In the case of observational studies, group assignments are generally made based on the preferences of the treating physicians or the patients. This creates a high potential for confounding (Section 2.3.A) because physicians and patients generally make decisions based on the condition of the patients. Although

---

[8] Ball, K., Berch, D.B., Helmers, K.F., et al. Effects of cognitive training interventions with older adults: a randomized controlled trial. *J. Am. Med. Assoc.* 2002; 288: 2271–81.

randomization can eliminate confounding, randomization will only work if it is unbiased.

To understand bias in treatment assignments, imagine the results if the investigators in the cognitive training study steered subjects with greater dementia into the cognitive training group because they believed the subjects really needed it. Or conversely, imagine the outcome if the investigators steered subjects away from the cognitive training group if they seemed too disorganized to benefit from it. Either way, the results of the study would be biased.

For this reason, it is essential that group assignment be made for each participant by someone with no contact with the participant using a random number table or a computer random number generator. Also, the assignments should be made at the time of enrollment, rather than prior to the enrollment, so that there is no chance that personnel change the order of enrollment into the study in order to influence the group assignment. In a well-funded multicenter trial these functions are performed by the coordinating center.

> **Tip**
>
> Group assignment should be done at the time of enrollment by someone with no contact with the participant using a random number table or generator.

Even with all of these controls, bias can occur. In the case of one multicenter study all of the above guidelines were followed and yet the system was tampered with. One of the research staff switched the assignments of respondents after they were made by the coordinating center so as to enable certain respondents to receive intensive counseling rather than standard of care. Since he always switched two respondents with different assignments it was hard to detect. (Had he only changed respondents to the active treatment arm the coordinating center would have caught the change because there would have been too many subjects in the intensive counseling arm.)

After the violation was found, the investigators changed the protocol such that the assignment of subjects by the coordinating center was done over a speakerphone so that both the subject and the staff member would hear which group the subject was being enrolled into. This prevented research staff from switching assignments (at least without the subject knowing it!).

I chose this example because when many people think of research malfeasance they think of investigators deliberately slanting things to make their research findings more compelling. In this case, the motive of the research assistant may have been the desire to provide intensive counseling to those subjects he felt needed it.

In an observational study, the investigators, the treating physicians, and the subjects usually know which treatment group the subject is part of. This creates a source of bias because the investigators, physicians, and subjects may have certain expectations based on what treatment the subject is receiving. For example, if an investigator knows that a subject is assigned to the treatment group, he or she may be inclined to see more improvement in the subject's symptoms than if the investigator knows the subject is assigned to the placebo group. Conversely, subjects who know that they are assigned to no treatment may be inclined to drop out of the study or feel that they are not improving.

In a randomized trial, bias due to the expectations of the investigators or the subjects can be eliminated through blinding (also referred to as masking). Blinding means preventing the investigator and/or the subject from knowing the treatment assignment.

When neither the investigator nor the subject knows what treatment the subject will be receiving, the trial is double-blinded. If only the investigator or the subject (but not both) is blinded to the assignment, the trial is single-blinded.

For randomized treatment trials blinding is usually done through the use of a placebo (an inactive substance) that is made to look and taste identically to the active treatment. Such trials are referred to as placebo-controlled trials. Typically, a pharmacist who has no contact with the subjects packages the treatments.

However, blinding of treatment assignment cannot always be accomplished. For example, in the case of the HIV prevention study discussed above, two different types of prevention interventions were being compared (multiple sessions of intensive counseling versus a few sessions of standard counseling). There was no way for participants or the study staff to be blinded as to which type of counseling participants were receiving.

In other cases, blinding may be possible but ethically problematic. To blind subjects and study staff to whether a surgical intervention had been performed requires performing a sham surgery. But it is debatable whether it is ethical to expose subjects to the risks of anesthesia without any benefit to them.[9]

Even when studies are blinded, it may be possible for subjects to learn their treatment assignments. For example, early drug treatment studies of HIV were blinded and placebo controlled; however, because some participants felt they would die if they did not receive treatment, they sent their pills to a commercial laboratory for testing. This led many investigators to conclude it was better to conduct open-label studies because blinded studies led to a systematic bias: patients who were doing poorly or who had some other way of getting the active drug were more likely to send their drugs for analysis.

Double-blinding is generally impossible with observational studies, although you may be able to have an evaluator who is blinded to treatment group assess each subject. There are a number of other sources of bias with observational studies, including selection and recall bias (with case–control studies) and ecologic bias (with ecologic studies). These are discussed in Section 2.6.

---

[9] Horng, S., Miller, F.G. Is placebo surgery unethical? *New Engl. J. Med.* 2002; 347: 137–9.

> **Definition**
>
> Blinding means preventing the investigator and/or the subject from knowing the treatment assignment.

> **Definition**
>
> When neither the investigator nor the subject knows what treatment the subject will be receiving, the trial is double-blinded. If only the investigator or the subject (but not both) is blinded to the assignment, the trial is single-blinded.

2.3.C Increasing generalizability

> Generalizability refers to the ability to apply the results of a study to populations other than the study sample.

> The results of a trial apply (generalize) only to populations that resemble the study sample.

> **Definition**
>
> Treatment efficacy is how well an intervention works in a research setting and treatment effectiveness is how well it works in a clinical setting.

> **Definition**
>
> Hawthorne effect refers to changes in participants' behavior due solely to their being observed.

Generalizability refers to the ability to apply the results of a study to populations other than the study sample. In general, the results of a trial only apply (generalize) to populations that resemble the study sample. For example, the results of a study performed on men may not generalize to women.

Although generalizability is an issue with both randomized and observational studies, it tends to be a greater problem with randomized studies because of the tremendous burdens placed on experimental subjects. They must agree to randomization and if the study is blinded, to not knowing what treatment they are taking. Also, most randomized studies require that subjects have frequent examinations and blood draws. The result is that randomized subjects are, by definition, different than the general population.

In addition, the conditions of randomized studies are different than the conditions of clinical practice. Experimental subjects tend to receive much more attention (e.g., education, counseling) than patients in normal practice. Therefore, you cannot assume that just because a treatment works under a tight research protocol it will work in clinical practice. For this reason, it's important to distinguish treatment efficacy (how well an intervention works in a research setting) from treatment effectiveness (how well an intervention works in a clinical setting).

Although observational studies more closely approximate treatment effectiveness than randomized studies, there still may be differences between observational trial participants and patients seen in purely clinical settings. Participants of observational studies may receive additional education or testing than patients would receive in standard clinical care. Finally, just observing participants may change their behavior. This is known as the Hawthorne effect.

2.3.D Length of time to conduct

Compared to randomized trials, observational studies are generally faster to conduct. This is especially true if you have an existing database or can use a case–control design (Section 2.6).

2.3.E Minimizing expense

Observational studies are generally less expensive than randomized studies especially if you have an existing database or can use a case–control design. Even when compared to prospective cohort designs (generally the most expensive observational design), randomized control trials are likely to be more expensive because when subjects are enrolled in a randomized study the study will be paying for all of the interventions (e.g., medicines, tests) associated with the trial. In an observational trial, the cost of the interventions is not generally paid by the study because the investigators are just "observing" the outcomes.

2.3.F Addressing a broader range of questions

Observational studies are generally able to answer a broader range of questions than randomized studies because there are many situations where it is unethical or impractical to randomize participants. For example, you cannot randomize persons to smoke or not to smoke. Also randomized control studies are rarely helpful in identifying the causes of disease outbreaks, such as food-borne illnesses.

2.3.G Empiric comparison of randomized and observational trials

Given the strengths and weaknesses of randomized controlled trials and observational studies, how do the results compare when they look at similar questions? Ioannidis and colleagues identified 45 topics in which randomized and non-randomized trials were performed.[10] They found that there was good correlation between the odds ratios produced by the two types of studies ($r = 0.75$; $P < 0.001$) with non-randomized studies tending to show larger treatment effects.

On the other hand, there have been some well-documented cases where randomized and non-randomized studies produced divergent results. For example, observational studies found lower rates of coronary artery disease among women taking hormone therapy than those not taking hormone treatment while a randomized trial found higher rates of coronary artery disease among women taking hormone therapy than those not taking hormone treatment and another trial found no difference in recurrent coronary artery events between those randomized to hormone treatment and those randomized to placebo.[11]

Overall, it makes sense to reserve the use of observational studies to instances where it is unethical or infeasible to perform a randomized controlled trial, or in cases when time is of the essence in obtaining a result. (Of course, there's never a rush to obtain the wrong answer.)

> Use observational designs when it is unethical or infeasible to perform a randomized controlled trial, or when time is of the essence in obtaining a result.

---

[10] Ioannidis, J.P.A., Haidich, A-B., Pappa, M., et al. Comparison of evidence of treatment effects in randomized and nonrandomized studies. *J. Am. Med. Assoc.* 2001; 286: 821–30.

[11] Grodstein, F., Clarkson, T.B., Manson, J.E. Understanding the divergent data on postmenopausal hormone therapy. *New Engl. J. Med.* 2003; 348; 645–50.

Table 2.3. Randomized study designs

	Description	Strengths	Weaknesses
Randomization of subjects to two or more groups	Each subject is randomly assigned to one of the study groups	Simplicity	None
Crossover design	Subjects are randomized to one group and then switched to the other group at a specified time	Increases power by allowing subjects to serve as their own control	The carryover effects of a treatment may make it difficult to ascribe successes or failures to the correct group
Factorial design	Subjects are randomized to more than one intervention	Answers two questions for (almost) the price of one	The efficiency of the design is lost if the interventions interact with one another

2.4 What are the different types of randomized controlled trials?

The three commonly used randomized-study designs, along with their strengths and weaknesses (compared to one another), are shown in Table 2.3.

2.4.A Randomization of subjects to two or more groups

Randomizing subjects to two or more groups is the most commonly used study design. It is simple and powerful.

2.4.B Crossover design

> With a crossover study, subjects are randomized to one group and then switched to the other group.

With crossover studies, subjects are randomized to one study arm and after a specified period of time are switched to the other arm. The design gives you two subjects for the price of one. Also, this design results in less variability than if you randomize subjects to different groups because crossover designs eliminate variability due to different subjects being in the different groups. With a crossover design, each subject serves as his or her own control, so there are no differences due to which subjects are randomized to which groups. Decreased variability results in increased power (Section 1.1). Crossover studies may also increase subject motivation because subjects will be guaranteed to receive the treatment (or both treatments) at least some of the time.

The major disadvantage of crossover studies is that they are subject to bias due to carryover effects. Carryover effects are due to the first treatment but occur during the second treatment.

For example, let's assume that you are studying the efficacy of antibiotic A versus antibiotic B in preventing infections. A particular subject is randomized to receive antibiotic A for 3 months and then to receive antibiotic B for the next 3 months. Now let's say the subject develops an infection in the fourth month. Does this represent a failure of antibiotic B to prevent the infection? Could it be that the infection occurred during the time that the patient was taking antibiotic A but did not manifest itself until the fourth month when the patient was already taking antibiotic B (carryover effect)? It would be very hard to know.

To mitigate this problem crossover studies should have a "washout" period, a time during which the subject does not receive either treatment. For example, Karst and colleagues studied the effect of the synthetic cannabinoid CT-3 on chronic neuropathic pain.[12] Patients were randomized to receive 7 days of treatment or placebo; after a 7-day washout they received the alternative assignment.

Although you can never be certain that you have eliminated bias due to carryover effects, crossover studies with sufficient washout periods are good designs when you cannot recruit enough subjects for a simple randomized study.

2.4.C Factorial studies

Factorial studies are designed to answer more than one question by randomizing each subject to more than one condition. For example, the Physicians' Health Study randomized subjects to (1) aspirin versus placebo for the prevention of cardiovascular disease; and (2) beta-carotene versus placebo for the prevention of cancer.[13] The major advantage of a factorial design is that you get two (or more) studies for the price of one.

Given this tremendous cost advantage, why don't investigators always use factorial designs? The problem with factorial designs is the possibility that the different conditions may affect one another (may interact).[14] For example, a potential

---

[12] Karst, M. Salim, K., Burstein, S., et al. Analgesic effect of the synthetic cannabinoid CT-3 on chronic neuropathic pain. *J. Am. Med. Assoc.* 2003; 290: 1757–62.

[13] The Steering Committee of the Physicians' Health Study Research Group. Final report on the aspirin component of the ongoing physicians' health study. *New Engl. J. Med.* 1989; 321: 129–35; Hennekens, C.H., Buring, J.E., Manson, J.E., et al. Lack of effect of long-term supplementation with beta-carotene on the incidence of malignant neoplasms and cardiovascular disease. *New Engl. J. Med.* 1996; 334: 1145–9.

[14] For a more detailed explanation of interactions see Katz, M.H. *Multivariable Analysis: A Practical Guide for Clinicians* (2nd edition). Cambridge: Cambridge University Press, 2005; pp. 11–13, 98–101, 134, 143–5.

Tip

Use factorial designs
only when you are sure
the two treatments
don't interact.

problem with the design of the Physicians' Health Study is that beta-carotene
may affect the incidence of cardiovascular disease.[15] You can, of course, check
for interactions when you perform factorial designs. However, it takes a larger
sample size to test for interactions (because you are essentially performing sub-
group analysis) so you will need to plan for a larger sample size, thereby losing
some of the cost savings in answering two questions at once.

2.5 What are the different methods of allocating subjects within a randomized design?

There are several different methods of allocating subjects within a randomized
design (Table 2.4).[16]

2.5.A Randomization with equal allocation

Randomization of an equal number of persons to each treatment group (simple
randomization) is the standard method of conducting a clinical experiment. It
is simple and it maximizes statistical power. Power is greatest when there are
equal numbers of subjects in each group.

Although randomization with equal allocation will result in *approximately*
equal numbers of subjects in each group one group may be bigger, by chance,
than another, just as if you flip a coin 10 times you will not necessarily get 5 heads
and 5 tails (Section 1.1). This can sometimes be a problem with small studies
(e.g., <20 subjects per group). Similarly, imbalances in prognostic characteristics
may also occur with simple randomization (e.g., subjects randomized to one
group may be significantly older than subjects randomized to a different group).

2.5.B Blocked randomization

If it is important to have exactly equal numbers of persons in each group, you
can perform a blocked randomization. Blocked randomization is usually performed in small blocks (e.g., 4 or 6 subjects). Assuming you have two groups, a
blocked randomization of 4 subjects will mean that 2 subjects will be in group
A and 2 subjects will be group B. Within the block assignment, the assignment
of subjects will be randomized.

---

[15] Morris, C.D., Carson, S. Routine vitamin supplementation to prevent cardiovascular disease:
a summary of the evidence for the US Preventive Services Task Force. *Ann. Intern. Med.* 2003;
139: 56–70.

[16] For a more detailed explanation of how to perform these different types of randomization, see
Friedman, L.M., Furberg, C.D., DeMets, D.L. *Fundamentals of Clinical Trials* (3rd edition). New York,
Springer, 1999.

Table 2.4. Different methods of random allocation

	Description	Strengths	Weaknesses
Randomization with equal allocation	Subjects have an equal likelihood of being randomized into each group	Maximizes power	Can result in imbalances in the number of subjects in each group and differences in baseline characteristics
Blocked randomization	Subjects are randomized in small blocks (e.g., 2, 4, or 6 subjects)	Assures an equal number of subjects in each group, may avoid confounding due to calendar time, study site	Easier for research personnel to predict the enrollment of a future subject
Randomization with unequal allocation	Subjects have a greater likelihood of being randomized into one group (usually the treatment arm) than another group (usually the placebo arm)	May help in recruiting subjects in cases where there are no existing treatments, may provide more information about the side effects of a new treatment	Less power than studies with an equal number of persons in each group; inconsistent with the principle of equipoise
Stratified randomization	Subjects are randomly allocated to the groups based on certain baseline characteristics	Prevents unequal distribution of important baseline characteristics	Requires knowledge of the important baseline characteristics prior to randomization; unworkable for more than a few baseline characteristics

Tip

Blocked randomization is only necessary with very small studies, when temporal changes are expected, or with multicenter studies.

In general, having an exactly equal number of subjects in each group is important only with very small studies. Two exceptions: larger studies where there are expected to be temporal changes affecting study enrollment and multicenter studies. If, for example, subjects enrolled early in a study are sicker than those enrolled in later years, and you get, by chance, a higher proportion of early enrollees in one group, than your comparisons may be biased. Similarly, with multicenter studies it may be important to avoid having an unequal proportion of subjects enrolled at different enrollment sites. These problems can be avoided with blocked randomization.

The major disadvantage of blocked randomization is that it is easier for study staff to figure out the assignment of a participant prior to enrollment (if the study is unblinded). Specifically, when you have enrolled all but the last subject of a block, the assignment of the last subject is predetermined (e.g., if you were randomizing subjects to group A and group B using a 4-subject block and the first three respondents were randomized as ABB, the fourth subject will be randomized to group A). This limitation can be overcome by randomly choosing among different size blocks (e.g., 2, 4, and 6 subjects) so that study staff members do not know the size of the block within which subjects are being randomized.

2.5.C Randomization with unequal allocation

> **Tip**
>
> Use randomization with unequal allocation as a participant incentive or when you are trying to learn more about the side effects of one arm of the study.

There are times when it is advantageous to randomize subjects in an unequal fashion such as a two-to-one randomization. For example, treatment trials of serious diseases (e.g., cancer or AIDS) may benefit from unequal allocation because subjects may be more motivated to participate if they have a greater than 50% chance of receiving the new treatment. Unequal randomizations may also be helpful in learning more about the side effects of a new treatment (because you can allocate more than half of the subjects to the new treatment group, you will have more data on the side effects of the drug).

> Equipoise exists when the research community believes that the different arms of the study are equal.

When it comes to study design, advantages bring disadvantages. With unequal randomization you lose power due to not having equal numbers of persons in each treatment group. With less power it is harder to reject the null hypothesis when it is false. In addition unequal allocation is inconsistent with the principle of equipoise. Equipoise refers to the belief of the investigator (or at least the research community) that the different arms of the study are equal. After all, if there is a clear indication that one arm is superior to the other it is unethical to randomize patients. Unequal allocation may give an implicit message that the investigator believes one arm is superior to the other.

2.5.D Stratified randomization

Stratified randomization is preferred when it is essential to have an equal distribution of baseline prognostic factors. Although randomization should produce study groups that are equal with respect to both observed and unobserved characteristics, sometimes, by chance, randomization produces two groups that differ on an important baseline characteristic, such as sex or age. For example, in a study comparing lung-volume-reduction surgery to medical therapy for severe emphysema more women were randomized to surgery than to medical therapy (42% versus 36%; $P = 0.04$).[17] Differences in baseline characteristics between the study groups such as occurred in this trial may confound the results of the study.

---

[17] National Emphysema Treatment Trial Research Group. A randomized trial comparing lung-volume-reduction surgery with medical therapy for severe emphysema. *New Engl. J. Med.* 2003; 348: 2059–73.

Stratified randomization assures an equal distribution of baseline characteristics between your study groups.

To avoid this problem, you can randomize persons within groups of important baseline characteristics (i.e., sex, age). This will ensure that you have an equal (or nearly equal) distribution of baseline characteristics between your study groups.

Another advantage of stratified randomization is that it may decrease the variability (i.e., the difference) between the two groups and thereby increase the power of your study.

In terms of which variables to stratify on, choose those that if unequally distributed in your study groups would result in doubts about the validity of your results. For example, Gallant and colleagues compared the efficacy of two anti-retroviral drugs, tenofovir and stavudine, in HIV-infected persons using a randomized double-blind design.[18] The randomization was stratified by HIV viral load ($<$ or $\geq$100,000 copies/ml) and CD4 count ($<$ or $\geq$200 cells). The reason for using a stratified-randomized design is that these two variables are so strongly associated with outcome, that if, by chance, simple randomization resulted in an unequal distribution of subjects on these two variables, the two randomized groups would not have been felt to be comparable.

Unfortunately it is not always clear prior to randomization which variables to stratify on. Also stratified randomization is unworkable if there are more than a few factors on which to stratify. If you have more than two or three baseline variables that are strongly associated with outcome, perform randomization with equal allocation and use multivariable analysis to statistically adjust for confounding in the analytic phase of your study (Chapter 6).

Tip

Consider stratified randomization if you have one or two baseline characteristics for which you must have an equal distribution in your study groups.

2.6 What are the different types of observational studies?

With observational studies the investigator assesses the participants without altering conditions (Section 2.3). As you can see in Table 2.5 there are several different types of observational studies.

The major difference between the first four types of observational studies listed in Table 2.5 – cross-sectional, prospective cohort, case–control, and nested case–control – is when the risk factors are measured in relation to the outcome. The fifth type – ecologic studies – are a special kind of observational study in that the observations are made at the aggregate level rather than at the individual subject level.

---

[18] Gallant, J.E., Staszewski, S., Pozniak, A.L., et al. Efficacy and safety of tenofovir df vs stavudine in combination therapy in antiretroviral-naïve patients. *J. Am. Med. Assoc.* 2004; 292: 191–201.

Table 2.5. Commonly used observational study designs

Type of observational study	When risk factors are measured	Advantages	Disadvantages
Cross-sectional	At the same time as the outcome	Determines prevalence	Weak evidence for causality
Prospective cohort	Prior to the outcome	Decreases likelihood that reverse causality is cause of association, eliminates recall bias, and determines incidence	Expensive, time consuming
Case–control	After the outcome	Efficient method for identifying cases (especially for uncommon diseases)	Selection bias (due to choice of controls and due to losses occurring before selection of cases and controls), and recall bias
Nested case–control	Prior to the outcome (testing of specimens may occur after outcome, but specimens are collected prior)	Efficient method for identifying cases and controls, minimizes recall bias	Requires foresight in the design of the prospective cohort
Ecologic study (aggregate data)	Varies	Allows study of broad social policy questions	Subject to the ecologic bias

2.6.A Cross-sectional studies

Definition

Prevalence is the *proportion* of individuals in a population who have a specific disease or condition at a particular moment in time.

Definition

Reverse causality is when the "effect" causes the "cause".

Cross-sectional studies are easy and fast to conduct because information is collected from subjects at a single point in time. Typically, cross-sectional studies are used to answer descriptive questions. For example: What is the prevalence of a disease in a community? Prevalence is the *proportion* of individuals in a population who have a specific disease or condition at a particular moment in time.

For example, Turner and colleagues conducted a cross-sectional of adults aged 18–35 years in Baltimore. They found that 8% of subjects had untreated gonococcal infection, chlamydial infection or both.[19] This is a very important finding because both gonorrhea and chlamydia have serious health consequences for the individual, are transmissible to others, and are easily curable.

Although cross-sectional studies are good for describing clinical phenomena like the prevalence of disease, they are not very good at answering analytic questions. The reason is that an association found in a cross-sectional study

---

[19] Turner, C.F., Rogers, S.M., Milleer, H.G., et al. Untreated gonococcal and chlamydial infection in a probability sample of adults. *J. Am. Med. Assoc.* 2002; 287: 726–33.

may go in either direction. The risk factor may cause the outcome (cause-effect) or the outcome may cause the risk factor (effect-cause, or reverse causality).

For example if a cross-sectional study finds a significant relationship between depression and alcohol abuse does this mean that depression causes alcoholism or that alcoholism causes depression? You can't tell (and neither can an alcoholic!)

On the other hand, in some instances reverse causality is an unlikely explanation. In such cases a cross-sectional study may satisfactorily answer an analytic question of whether or not an association exists. For example, a cross-sectional study found that smokers were more likely to have facial wrinkles than non-smokers.[20] Although from the statistical association it is equally likely that facial wrinkles cause smoking as smoking causes facial wrinkles, it is very unlikely that people begin to smoke because they have facial wrinkles. As always, common sense is the most important technique for understanding statistical associations!

Cross-sectional studies are also very helpful for determining the frequency of risk behaviors, which can be very useful in estimating sample sizes for analytic studies (Chapter 7).

2.6.B Prospective cohort studies

In a prospective cohort study the sample is assembled prior to the development of the outcome and followed over time. At entry into the study, subjects are assessed for exposures of interest and evaluated to make sure that they do not already have the outcome being studied.

Compared to cross-sectional designs, prospective studies provide much stronger evidence in support of a causal relationship. The reason is that by measuring the risk factor ahead of the outcome you reduce the possibility that the "effect" causes the "cause" (reverse causality).

> Prospective studies are the strongest observational design for supporting causality.

Since information about risk factors is collected ahead of the development of disease, prospective studies also minimize recall bias. Recall bias is especially a problem with case–control studies (Section 2.6.C) because developing a disease may make it more likely that subjects will remember an exposure. Since prospective studies minimize the likelihood that reverse causality is the cause of an association and decrease recall bias, they are the strongest observational design for supporting causality.

> **Definition**
>
> Incidence rate is the number of new cases of a particular condition in an at-risk population per unit time.

While cross-sectional studies can be used to calculate prevalence, only prospective studies can be used to calculate incidence rate. Incidence rate is the number of new cases of a particular condition in an at-risk population per unit time (Section 4.6).

---

[20] Ernster, V.L., Grady, D., Miike, R., et al. Facial wrinkling in men and women, by smoking status. *Am. J. Public Health* 1995; 85: 78–82.

The length of follow-up time for a longitudinal study is determined based on how long it takes to develop the disease (as well as the length of time for which the investigators can get research funding!).

The Framingham Heart Study, the most famous prospective cohort study ever assembled has been following 5209 men and women from Framingham Massachusetts since 1948. The study has been such a success in identifying the predictors of cardiac disease that 5124 children of the original cohort members and their spouses were enrolled in the Framingham Offspring Study in 1971 and their grandchildren were enrolled in 2001.

A major disadvantage of prospective cohort studies is that they take a long time to perform, especially if the disease develops slowly. This makes them costly and inefficient for studying uncommon diseases (because few persons will develop the disease even in a large cohort). Long observation periods also introduce bias due to subjects being lost to follow-up. With long follow-up periods temporal changes (e.g., introduction of new treatments, change in clinical practices) may influence your results. Finally, with a prospective cohort design you run the risk that the answer to your question may be less relevant (or already answered!) by the time your study is complete.

2.6.C Case–control studies

> **Tip**
>
> Use a case–control design to study uncommon diseases.

In a case–control study the subjects are assembled based on whether they have experienced the outcome (cases) or not (controls). Once the cases and controls are identified, the frequencies of the different risk factors for the disease are compared between the cases and controls.

The major advantage of case–control studies is that they are a very efficient study design, especially for studying uncommon diseases.

For example, Forsyth and colleagues used a case–control study to assess whether aspirin use in the setting of viral illness among children is associated with Reye's syndrome, a deadly disease.[21] Since Reye's syndrome is rare, a surveillance system was set up in 108 hospitals from 32 states within the USA and 20 hospitals in Canada. Over an 18-month period only 24 cases were identified. These cases were matched to 48 controls. The controls were children with an antecedent illness who did not have Reye's syndrome. Although the total number of cases was small, the study produced dramatic results: 88% of case subjects and 17% of controls had received aspirin prior to the onset of Reye's syndrome (matched odds ratio = 35; 95% confidence intervals, 4.2–288).

---

[21] Forsyth, B.W., Horwitz, R.I., Acampora, D., et al. New epidemiologic evidence confirming that bias does not explain the aspirin/Reye's syndrome association. *J. Am. Med. Assoc.* 1989; 261: 2517–24.

For case–control methodology to be valid, the cases and controls must originate from the same population. This is the reason that Forsyth and colleagues recruited controls from the medical practices of physicians with the same specialty (e.g., pediatrics, family practice) located in the same area as each case subject. Cases and controls were also matched based on whether or not they had visited a physician for their illness.

However, it is sometimes hard to prove whether the cases and the controls are from the same population. For this assumption to be true in the case of Forsyth and colleagues study, the controls seen in these medical practices would have had to been hospitalized in one of the surveillance hospitals if they had developed Reye's syndrome. If the controls are not selected from the same population as the cases, then the results of the study will be biased.

Since cases and controls are chosen after the development of the outcome, case–control studies may suffer from another form of selection bias: loss of cases and/or controls prior to their selection. For example, if some potential cases die prior to the assembly of the cases, then your sample of cases is not fully representative of the population of cases.

Besides selection bias, case–control studies may be biased by participant recall. This is particularly a problem if cases are more (or less) likely to remember an exposure than controls. For example, people with cancer may be more likely to report prior exposures than persons without cancer because the cancer has caused them to examine their life more closely for an explanation as to why they became ill. On the other hand, some exposures may have been written down in medical charts prior to development of the condition, or be factors that do not change (e.g., genetic factors).

Case–control studies can be matched or unmatched.[22] There are two types of matching: individual matching and frequency matching. With individual matching each case is individually matched (linked) with one or more controls. With frequency matching, controls are matched to cases as a group such that the distribution of the cases and controls on each strata of the matched variable is similar. For example, let's say you wanted to match on age. With individual matching, you would match a 45-year-old case with a 45-year-old control (plus or minus some range, say 5 years). With frequency matching, you would first need to know the distribution of cases on each strata of age. If 15% of cases were between the ages of 40 and 50 years, you would choose controls such that 15% would be between the ages of 40 and 50 years.

---

[22] Prospective cohort studies can also be matched. However, you will rarely see matched prospective cohort studies because it is generally better to deal with confounding in a cohort study using stratification or multivariable modeling.

The advantage of matching is that you eliminate confounding due to those variables that you match on. Another advantage is that you assure that the distribution of cases and controls on matching variables is sufficiently similar that you can use stratification or multivariable analysis in order to eliminate confounding. This is especially important with multiple category nominal independent variables (e.g., type of cancer, type of pre-existing disease). In the absence of matching, you may not be able to adjust for a multiple category nominal variable because there is insufficient overlap between the cases and the controls (e.g., there are ten cases with a history of breast cancer but no controls with a history of breast cancer, there are 15 controls with diabetes but only one case with diabetes, etc.).

A disadvantage of matching is that it increases the difficulty (and cost!) of identifying controls (this is particularly a problem if there are a limited number of potential controls). Also, once you match for a variable, you cannot study the impact of that variable on the outcome. This is not a problem if the relationship between the potential confounder and the outcome has already been well established. For example, if you were studying the impact of diesel fumes on lung cancer you wouldn't lose information by matching on smoking status because the relationship of smoking to lung cancer is already well documented. Finally, if the variables that you match for are associated with the exposure, then matching may introduce selection bias into your study.

Individually matched data must be analysed with specialized statistics that take into account the individual linking of cases (Section 5.11). Frequency matched data can be analysed as you would unmatched data but you must adjust for the strata that you have matched on using stratified or multivariable analysis.

Considering the advantages and disadvantages of matching, in general, it is best to avoid matching. An exception would be small studies (say under 50 subjects) where you will have difficulty statistically adjusting for all possible confounders unless you match. With larger studies, you also may need to match if you have multiple category nominal independent variables.[23]

Having identified the pool for your controls and whether or not to match, you need to decide how many controls per case to enroll. The greatest study efficiency

> **Tip**
>
> Perform matched studies with very small sample sizes or when you have multiple category nominal variables.

---

[23] Matching is a very complicated topic. However, because my general advice is to avoid it, I have kept the discussion on matching brief. Readers who are interested in understanding the implications of matching better should see the following references, from which I drew much of the above discussion: Rothman, K.J., Greenland, S. *Modern Epidemiology* (2nd edition). Philadelphia, PA: Lippincott Williams & Wilkins, 1998, pp. 147–61; Kelsey, J.L., Whittemore, A.S., Evans, A.S., Thompson, W.D. *Methods in Observational Epidemiology* (2nd edition). Oxford: Oxford University Press, 1996, pp. 214–39; Szklo, M., Nieto, F.J. *Epidemiology: Beyond the Basics.* Gaithersburg, Maryland: Aspen Publication, pp. 40–8.

(in terms of information per subject) occurs when you have an equal number of cases and controls. But sometimes, such as with rare conditions, it is much easier to obtain controls than cases. When you can't obtain enough cases to answer your research question using a one-to-one match, you can increase the power of your study by adding additional controls. The gain in power with additional controls levels off at about four controls per case.

For example, Meier and colleagues conducted a case–control study assessing the association between antibiotic use and risk of subsequent acute myocardial infarction.[24] (The underlying hypothesis is that bacterial infections may be an underlying cause of coronary artery disease.) The investigators identified 3315 patients from the computerized patient records of 350 general practices in the UK. They matched each case with four controls. Cases and controls were matched on age, sex, general practice attended, and calendar time. Using a matched multivariable analysis that adjusted for potential confounders, they found that cases were significantly less likely to have used tetracycline antibiotics (OR = 0.70, 95% CI, 0.55–0.90) and quinolones (OR = 0.45; 95% CI, 0.21–0.95) than controls. Had they not matched each case with four controls, they may not have had sufficient power to demonstrate a statistically significant association between antibiotic use and myocardial infarction.

> Case–control studies cannot be used for determining the prevalence or incidence of a disease.

An important limitation of case–control studies is that they cannot be used for determining the prevalence or incidence of a disease. This is because the subjects are chosen on the basis of whether or not they have the disease.

2.6.D Nested case–control studies

A nested case–control study is a case–control study where the cases and controls are drawn from the subjects enrolled in a prospective cohort study. It has several advantages over a traditional case–control study. Since cases and controls are chosen from the same cohort, there can be no question that the cases and controls are drawn from the same population. Also because of the prospective nature of the cohort, information on risk factors and potential confounders has been collected prior to the development of the disease, eliminating recall bias.

For example, a nested case–control study turned out to be an excellent design for determining whether the long-chain n − 3 polyunsaturated fatty acids found in fish decrease the risk of sudden death among healthy persons. Before explaining their design and results, let's consider some other study designs to answer this question.

---

[24] Meier, C.R., Derby, L.E., Jick, S.S., Vasiolakis, C., Jick, H. Antibiotics and risk of subsequent first-time acute myocardial infarction. *J. Am. Med. Assoc.* 1999; 281: 427–31.

Let's say you want to answer this question using a traditional case–control study. You have a major problem: you can't interview dead people about their fish eating habits (or much else for that matter!). You could interview their family members about the decedent's fish eating consumption but how accurately would family members remember their relative's fish eating habits? Would they know the type of fish (not all fish have the same amount of long-chain polyunsaturated fatty acids) and the size of the portion? Probably not! Also, the memories of family members might be colored by their loss of a relative to sudden death and their knowledge that eating fish is good for the heart.

Having abandoned a case–control model, you consider a prospective cohort study (observational or randomized). However your sample size calculations shows you that you would need a huge sample size and a very long follow-up period because the incidence of sudden death among healthy individuals is extremely low (<0.001 cases per year). (Said a different way, if you followed 5000 people for 5 years fewer than 25 cases would experience sudden death.)

In contrast to the problems in performing a case–control or a prospective cohort study, Albert and colleagues answered this question elegantly, quickly, and cheaply using a nested case–control design.[25] The prospective cohort was the Physicians' Health Study; it was initially assembled for a randomized crossover trial evaluating aspirin and beta-carotene in the prevention of coronary artery disease and cancer (Section 2.4.C). The investigators took advantage of the large sample size, the long follow-up of members of this cohort, and most importantly, the foresight of the original investigators to collect blood specimens from the participants.

Of the 22,071 male physicians enrolled in the study, 201 had sudden death within 17 years of study follow-up. Of these 201 physicians, 119 had an adequate blood specimen banked at the start of the study, and 94 of these were free of confirmed cardiovascular disease before death. These 94 persons were matched with two controls from the cohort who were alive, free of confirmed cardiovascular disease at the time of case ascertainment, and had an adequate blood specimen.

Compared to men whose blood levels of long-chain $n-3$ polyunsaturated fatty acids were in the lowest quartile, the adjusted relative risk of death among those in the highest quartile was 0.19 (95% CI, 0.05–0.71), suggesting that long-chain $n-3$ polyunsaturated fatty acids have a preventive effect on sudden death.

Nested case–control studies are particularly efficient when subjects must be tested on a expensive or difficult to perform assay. In the case of this study, the

---

[25] Albert, C.M., Campos, H., Stampfer, M.J., et al. Blood levels of long-chain $n-3$ fatty acids and the risk of sudden death. *New Engl. J. Med.* 2002; 345: 1113–18.

investigators only had to determine long-chain n − 3 polyunsaturated fatty acids levels for 282 participants (94 cases + 188 controls), rather than the 22, 071 participants originally enrolled.

Tip

When initiating prospective cohorts, bank serum and cells.

The major limitation of the nested case–control study is that the design is not viable unless information about the risk factor or a specimen was collected at the beginning of the study. For example, if the investigators of the Physicians' Health Study hadn't the foresight to bank serum, a nested case–control design would not have been a viable design to assess the relationship between long-chain n − 3 polyunsaturated fatty acids and sudden death. Therefore, if you ever perform a prospective cohort study bank serum (and also cells) that can be used for future work. Another potential disadvantage of the nested-case–control is that not all tests can be performed on stored specimens; in some cases, stored specimens may produce different results than if the test were performed on a fresh specimen.

With regard to matching cases and controls, and the optimal number of controls per case, the same considerations hold for nested case–control studies as for traditional case–control studies.

2.6.E Ecologic studies

Definition

Ecologic studies collect data at the aggregate level.

Ecologic studies collect data in the aggregate rather than at the individual level. Data may be collected at the level of a neighborhood, a city, a state, or a country.

Ecologic studies are generally used when data do not exist on an individual level or when the primary focus is the well-being of an entire community rather than that of the individuals within the community.

For example, Cohen and colleagues looked at the impact of boarded-up housing on rates of gonorrhea in 107 cities.[26] They found that cities with a higher percentage of boarded-up housing had higher rates of gonorrhea. Their results are consistent with the hypothesis that physical deterioration of neighborhoods leads to social isolation and unsafe health practices.

Definition

The ecologic fallacy is an incorrect conclusion about individual behavior based on aggregate data.

Although their data are compelling, it is important to note that Cohen and colleagues have not collected any data from individuals. Therefore it is possible that none of the cases of gonorrhea occurred among persons living in neighborhoods with boarded-up buildings and that their findings are confounded by some other factor. An incorrect conclusion about individual behavior based on aggregate data is referred to as the ecologic fallacy.

---

[26] Cohen, D.A., Mason, K., Bedimo, A., et al. Neighborhood physical conditions and health. *Am. J. Public Health* 2003; 93: 467–71.

Table 2.6. Study hypotheses

Hypothesis	Prototype	Example
Null	There will be no association between the *risk factor* and the *outcome* among the *study sample*	There will be no association between *exercise fitness* and *coronary artery disease* among *community dwelling persons over 65 years of age*
Alternative	There will be an association between the *risk factor* and the *outcome* among the *study sample*	There will be an association between *exercise fitness* and *coronary artery disease* among *community dwelling persons over 65 years of age*

Strategies for minimizing the ecologic fallacy exist.[27] However, you can never completely eliminate this bias and for that reason ecologic studies are best used to generate hypotheses that can be tested using other study designs.

2.7 Do I need to specify a particular hypothesis for my study?

Yes. If you are performing an analytic study it is important to specify the study hypothesis – what you are hoping to prove – prior to undertaking data collection.

The study hypothesis should be stated in both the null form (there is *no* difference) and the alternative form (there is a difference) (Table 2.6). Note that the alternative hypothesis, both the prototype and the example are stated in a neutral way (without direction). This is referred to as a two-sided hypothesis.

The reason that you need to state both a null and an alternative hypothesis is that statistical analysis is based on inferential reasoning (Section 1.1). We take a sample of a population and using a variety of statistical tests assess the probability that an association found in a sample could have occurred by chance if there were no true association in the population.[28] If the probability that the association could have occurred by chance falls below our pre-specified threshold (usually $P < 0.05$), we reject the null hypothesis (i.e., that there is no true association in the population) and consider the alternative hypothesis (i.e., that there is a true association in the population).

Of course, just because the probability of getting a particular result due to chance is <0.05, doesn't mean that it is impossible (in fact, statistically a result that occurs at a probability of 0.05 will occur once in 20 times). Concluding that there

---

[27] King, G. *A Solution to the Ecological Inference Problem*. Princeton: Princeton University Press, 1997.
[28] I am assuming that we are trying to disprove the null hypothesis. The process for trying to "prove" the null hypothesis is true is different. See equivalence studies in Section 7.11.

is a true association between two variables when the association is really due to chance (falsely rejecting the null hypothesis) is referred to as a type I error.

2.8 Can I specify an alternative hypothesis with a specific direction?

Yes. Indeed there are advantages to stating and testing one-sided hypotheses. In particular, it is easier to detect a statistical association when you specify a one-sided hypothesis (easier in the sense that it can be established with a smaller sample size for a given effect size or a smaller effect size for a given sample size). However, one-sided hypotheses can be used only on the rare occasions when only one side of the alternative hypothesis is possible or important.

For example, Hodnett and colleagues randomized women in labor to receive either usual care or continuous labor support by specially trained nurses.[29] The alternative hypothesis was that receiving labor support would result in a reduction in the Cesarean section rate. The rationale for testing a one-sided hypothesis was that there was no theoretical or empirical basis for why providing labor support would be harmful compared to usual care. Also, from a practical point of view, showing that nurses were harmful and they provided no benefit would have the same implication (keep to standard of care). Therefore, the only meaningful result would be that nurses were beneficial. Using a one-tailed test (hypotheses have "sides" and tests have "tails") they found that nurse support did not decrease Cesarean section rates compared to usual care.

I cannot emphasize enough how infrequently it is appropriate to test one-sided hypotheses. To illustrate why, consider the case of a study designed to test the effect of folate therapy on restenosis following coronary-stent placement.[30] Folate therapy is known to lower homocysteine levels. Elevated homocysteine levels are a risk factor for coronary artery disease and are associated with higher rates of restenosis. A prior randomized study had found that patients who received folate had significantly reduced rates of restenosis following angioplasty.[31] In their double-blind, placebo-controlled randomized trial the investigators found that the rate of restenosis was **higher** among persons who received folate. Although there was uncertainty as to whether folate worked, no one expected prior to this study that it would increase the rate of restenosis.

---

[29] Hodnet, E.D., Lowe, N.K., Hannah, M.E., et al. Effectiveness of nurses as providers of birth labor support in North American hospitals. *J. Am. Med. Assoc.* 2002; 288: 1373–81.

[30] Lange, H., Suryapranata, H., De Luca, G., et al. Folate therapy and in-stent restenosis after coronary stenting. *New Engl. J. Med.* 2004; 350: 2673–81.

[31] Schnyder, G., Roffi, M., Pin, R., et al. Decreased rate of coronary restenosis after lowering of plasma homocysteine levels. *New Engl. J. Med.* 2001; 345: 1593–600.

Therefore, even if one side of the hypothesis seems very unlikely, always use a two-tailed tests.

This does not mean that you can't have an opinion about which direction the findings will go. Most of us do. But for statistical testing two-sided hypotheses are a more rigorous standard and what most journal reviewers will expect.

2.9 Can my study have more than one question?

Absolutely. In fact, I recommend it. Recruiting subjects, interviewing them, reviewing medical records, and cleaning data sets are all time consuming activities. If you can design your study so that you can answer more than one question your study will be more efficient.

To answer more than one question you need to collect data on more than one outcome. (Collecting data on additional risk factors for the same outcome does not usually lead to answering multiple questions because the additional risk factors address the same question: What causes the outcome?)

Multiple outcomes may represent different stages of the same disease process. For example, a study of the impact of smoking on heart disease might collect data on the occurrence of angina, myocardial infarction, and death. If smoking causes coronary artery disease you would expect it to increase the occurrence of all three outcomes. The fact that it does strengthens the causal explanation.

Multiple outcomes may also represent different disease processes influenced by the same risk factors. For example, studies of the effect of hormone use in postmenopausal women have collected data on the outcomes of bone fractures, coronary artery disease, and dementia.

Finally, it may be beneficial to collect data on multiple outcomes that are unrelated to one another. For example, the HIV Cost and Services Utilization Study (HCSUS) was a nationally representative sample of persons receiving care for HIV. Since it required population-based sampling of a low prevalence, highly confidential condition it was extremely difficult and expensive to recruit the sample.[32] However, once recruited, the only limitation to how much data could be collected was the patience and stamina of the respondents.

The HCSUS baseline interview included questions on a number of diverse risk factors and outcomes and took over an hour to complete. The two follow-up interviews were a little shorter because they did not have to capture data on basic demographics. The result was that the investigators performed a variety of

---

[32] Frankel, M.R., Shapiro, M.F., Duan, N., et al. National probability samples in studies of low-prevalence diseases. Part II: Designing and implementing the HIV cost and services utilization sample. *Health Serv. Res.* 1999; 34: 969–92.

Table 2.7. Different types of variables

Type of variable	Description of variable	Examples
Interval (continuous)	Equal sized intervals on all parts of the scale are equal	Blood pressure, age, temperature
Categorical variables		
Dichotomous	Two categories	Yes/no, alive/dead
Ordinal	Multiple categories that can be ordered	NYHA classification for heart failure, stage of cancer
Nominal	Multiple categories that cannot be ordered	Ethnicity, type of cancer, cause of death

analyses on a diverse set of topics including receipt of medical care, use of anti-retroviral medications, prevalence of mental illness, prevalence of alcohol consumption, unmet need for dental care, and case management.

2.10 What kind of measures should I use?

The different types of measures (variables) are shown in Table 2.7.

With an interval (also called continuous) variable (e.g., cholesterol) equal sized differences (intervals) on all parts of the scale are equal. Blood pressure is an interval variable because the difference between a blood pressure of 180 and 183 (3 mmHg) is the same as the difference between a blood pressure of 280 and 283 (3 mmHg). Since there are multiple points on an interval scale, interval variables are rich in information.

In comparison, dichotomous variables (the simplest kind of categorical variable) have only two possible variables, such as "yes" or "no" and therefore provide less information. This is easy to appreciate clinically: a cholesterol level of 240 mg/dl and of 340 mg/dl would both be coded as "yes" for a variable "elevated cholesterol", but you would be much more concerned about a patient with a cholesterol of 340 mg/dl.

Since interval variables have more information, it is better to collect information in this form. Also, while it is easy to turn an interval variable into a dichotomous variable by simply choosing a cut-off, the reverse is impossible.

As the name implies, ordinal variables are categorical variables with multiple categories that can be ordered, but for which there is not a fixed interval between the categories. An example of an ordinal variable is the New York Heart Association (NYHA) Classification for Heart Failure.[33] It classifies a patient's function into 1 of 4 classes as shown in Table 2.8.

---

[33] http://www.bcbst.com/MPManual/New_York_Association_(NYHA)_Classification.htm

Table 2.8. New York Heart Association (NYHA) Classification for Heart Failure

NYHA class	Exercise tolerance	Symptoms
I	No limitation	No symptoms during usual activity
II	Mild limitation	Comfortable with rest or with mild exertion
III	Moderate limitation	Comfortable only at rest
IV	Severe limitation	Any physical activity brings on discomfort and symptoms occur at rest

> **Definition**
>
> Ordinal variables are categorical variables with multiple categories that can be ordered, but for which there is not a fixed interval between the categories.

> **Definition**
>
> Nominal variables are categorical variables with multiple categories that cannot be ordered.

As you go from classes I–IV heart failure worsens, but the degree of worsening as you go from one class to the next is not equal.

Ordinal variables provide less information than interval variables, but more than nominal variables (discussed below). Depending on how many categories there are (more is better), the sample size (more is better) and the distribution of the variable (Section 4.2 and 5.8) ordinal variables may sometimes be treated as interval variables in statistical analyses. Alternatively they can be analysed using non-parametric statistics (Section 5.4).

Nominal variables are categorical variables with multiple categories that cannot be ordered. An example of a nominal variable is ethnicity. In the USA, the variable is usually represented as White/Caucasian; African-American, Latino, Asian and Pacific Islanders, Native-American/Eskimo or other. Of course, if you want greater specificity you can distinguish the categories further; for example, there are over 15 distinct ethnicities that comprise the group Asian and Pacific Islander category. Regardless of the number of categories, there is no sensible ordering of the categories. Although we usually assign numbers for each category (e.g., 1 = White/Caucasian, 2 = African-American, etc.) to enter the data into the computer, the numbers have no arithmetic meaning.

2.11 How many subjects will I need for my study?

"How many subjects will I need for my study?" is probably the most frequently asked question by investigators planning a study. And for good reason. If you do not have enough subjects, then no matter how perfect your study design you will not be able to answer your question.

Sample size calculations must be performed prior to the collection and analysis of your data. Nonetheless, I will defer the discussion of this topic until Chapter 7 after we have reviewed the different types of statistical analyses available. The reason is that you need to know what statistical test you will be using in order to be able to perform a power calculation.

2.12 How do I obtain an institutional review board approval to perform a research study?

A critical step for performing any study involving human subjects is to have the protocol approved by an institutional review board (IRB); these boards are also referred to as human subjects committees.

The purpose of an IRB is to review research protocols to make sure that the rights of research subjects are protected. This includes being sure that the subjects are fully informed and have consented to participate in the study, that the risks are reasonable, that confidentiality is maintained, and that the study will create new knowledge (because no risk to a subject is reasonable without the promise of new knowledge).

Almost all universities, many hospitals, federal agencies (e.g., the CDC), local governments, and some community groups have an IRB to facilitate research. IRB members should be a mix of researchers, clinicians, lawyers, ethicists, and community members. Although all IRBs must operate within federal regulations, each one has it's own procedures. Therefore, it is best to determine what IRB you will be using and request information from them on protocol submission.[34]

---

[34] For a review of human subjects issues see: Rozovsky, R.A., Adams, R.K. *Clinical Trials and Human Research: A Practical Guide to Regulatory Compliance.* San Francisco, CA: Jossey-Bass, 2003.

Data management

3.1 How do I manage my data?

The procedures for collecting, entering, cleaning, and recoding data as well as deriving variables and exporting data are shown schematically in Figure 3.1 and explained in this chapter.

3.2 What procedures should I follow in collecting data?

Armed with your research question and study design, you are ready to plan your data collection. As you make your decisions document them in your study manual.

Information that should be included in a study manual includes:

- How subjects will be enrolled
  - Sites (e.g., how sites were selected, why sites that met selection criteria were excluded)
  - Inclusion criteria (e.g., eligibility criteria, such as age, residence, health status)
  - Exclusion criteria (e.g., inability to speak certain languages, dementia)
  - Sampling scheme (e.g., consecutive patients, convenience sample)
- Time period of study
  - Date of start of enrollment
  - Date enrollment is (scheduled to be) completed
  - Date at which follow-up will be terminated
- Methods by which data will be collected
  - Questionnaires, interviews, record reviews, electronic download of data, etc.
- Methods by which data will be entered
  - Single entry, double entry by same person, double entry by different people, etc.
  - Software package used for data entry (e.g., Epi info, EpiData, etc.).

Your manual should be as detailed as possible. A good study manual will protect against bias and make it a breeze to write the methods section of your paper. If there are unavoidable changes in your procedures as you perform your study

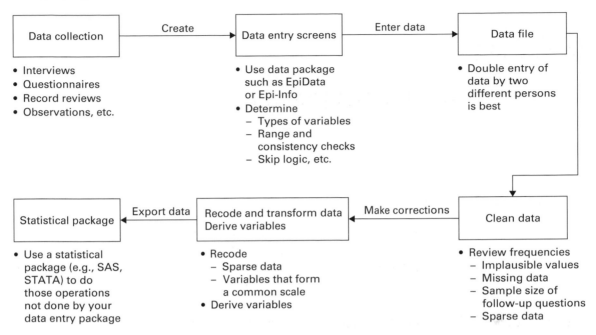

Figure 3.1   Data management process.

(e.g., elimination of a study site) document these as well.[35] Include as an appendix to your study manual your data collection instruments, institutional review board (IRB) forms, protocols for training study staff, decision rules on coding surveys, and other written materials you develop. Be sure to include dates with your materials so you will know what happened when.

3.3 How do I create data collection instruments?

By this point in the process, you will know whether you will be collecting your data via questionnaires, interviews, medical record reviews, download of existing data, another method, or a combination of methods.[36]

Unless you are downloading existing data, you will need a form on which to collect the data. The form will be paper or (increasingly) a computerized screen.

There are many advantages to collecting data directly onto the computer. It saves the time and expense of a separate data entry process and eliminates errors that can creep into your data when you enter them onto a computer from a paper form.

---

[35] For more on study procedures, see: Friedman, L.M., Furberg, C.D., DeMets, D.L. *Fundamentals of Clinical Trials* (3rd edition). New York: Springer, 1999.

[36] For detailed advice on developing questionnaires, interview protocols, and other forms of data collection see: Kelsey, J.L., Whittemore, A.S., Evans, A.S., Thompson, W.D. *Methods in Observational Epidemiology* (2nd edition). Oxford: Oxford University Press, 1996, pp. 364–412.

Tip

If possible, collect your data directly on a computer instead of using paper forms.

In the case of interview studies, it is possible to design computerized data collection forms such that the computer will tell the interviewer in real time that an implausible value has been entered, that a question has been missed, or that the answer to a question is inconsistent with the answer to another question on the survey. This then allows the interviewer to obtain the correct data prior to completing the interview. Computerized data entry also works well for medical record reviews where the reviewer can enter the abstracted data directly from the record into the computer.

For advice on choosing a data entry program along with more information on range checks, skip logic, and consistency checks, see Section 3.4.

Computerizing data collection instruments is not always feasible with questionnaires. For example, you will need to use paper questionnaires if you are doing a survey by mail. Similarly, if you are having multiple subjects completing the questionnaire at one time (e.g., in a classroom setting), you may not be able to afford enough computers to let each subject use one.

In considering the use of computerized questionnaires, you must also consider the computer literacy of your subjects. Many people are frightened by computers. On the other hand, some subjects may respond more honestly to sensitive questions, if they can input their answers directly into the computer rather than having to tell an interviewer.[37]

If you must collect the data on paper, consider designing the data collection forms so that they can be scanned directly into the computer. This will minimize errors due to data entry. Unfortunately scanning does not work well with write-in responses.

Finally, if it is impossible to collect the data directly on the computer or on scannable forms, design your paper entry forms to facilitate accurate date entry. Use a single box or underscore for each letter or number of the response. If possible, place the responses to the questions in a straight line down the right hand side of the page so the operator is not forced to scan the whole page looking for the data to enter.

Whether your data collection instrument is paper, computerized, or scannable, you will need to make some basic determinations about the data you will be collecting including the variable types and the acceptable responses for each variable.

3.3.A Types of variables and responses

One of the major tasks in the creation of your data entry instruments is to specify the variable types and the potential response to each one.

---

[37] Kissinger, P., Rice, J., Farley, T., et al. Application of computer-assisted interviews to sexual behavior research. *Am. J. Epidemiol.* 1999; 149: 950–4.

Types of commonly used variables:
- Unique identification (ID) number
- Numeric
- Logic (Yes/No)
- Date
- Text

Each subject must have a unique ID number. Most data entry programs will automatically assign consecutive numbers to your subjects as you enter the data.

Numeric variables may be whole numbers or decimals. If you anticipate decimals, specify how many digits you will accept to the right of the decimal place (e.g., one decimal place (e.g., 1.2) or two decimal places (e.g., 1.26), or three decimal places (e.g., 1.264), etc.). This will help avoid data entry errors.

A numeric variable type may be used for an *interval variable* such as systolic blood pressure and an *ordinal variable* such as the New York Heart Association Classification for Heart Failure, or a *categorical variable* such as ethnicity. With a categorical variable you will assign numbers to the different categories (e.g., 1 = African-American, 2 = Caucasian, 3 = Latino, etc.) even though the numbers have no numeric meaning. On the data collection form the numbers should appear, in small but legible font, next to the box or underscore denoting the category.

For your numeric variables, specify the range of acceptable values (i.e., a systolic blood pressure of 180 mmHg is high, but a systolic blood pressure of 810 mmHg is inconsistent with life). Once specified, your data entry programs can automatically decline values that are outside the range of plausible values (Section 3.4).

Logic variables are entered as yes or no. For some types of analysis it may be necessary to recode the variable to a numeric value later, but for the sake of data entry, especially if the interviewer or the subject is directly entering the data, fewer mistakes will be made if the questions are answered as "yes/no" rather than "1/0".

Date variables are used for specifying variables such as date of birth, enrollment date. In the analysis phase, statistical programs will automatically determine the interval between any two dates. Therefore, it is best to collect the dates that events occurred, rather than having the respondent or interviewer determine the interval between them.

Text variables allow you to enter open-ended comments made by subjects. Remember, however, that text responses cannot be analysed statistically unless you categorize certain responses with numbers (e.g., code as "1" if respondent mentions time as a reason for not getting a mammogram; code as "2" if respondent mentions money as a reason for not getting a mammogram). Nonetheless, if there is any chance you will want to analyse this data, it is easier to do so if you

Tip

Collect the dates that events occurred rather than the intervals between the events.

Tip

Use text variables to enter open-ended responses only if you will be coding them numerically later.

have entered it into your data entry program rather than if you try to go back later to the paper form or a recording of the interview.

If you do not intend to analyse text data, but want a record of the comments made by your respondents, it may be easier to enter the responses in a word processing program. This will save you from creating an unusually large data file, which can sometimes slow data analysis.

3.3.B Naming variables

> **Tip**
>
> In naming your variables, use the full name or a common abbreviation, when possible.

> **Tip**
>
> If you have several variables measuring the same construct over time use consecutive numbers to name the variables.

> **Definition**
>
> Value labels are descriptions of the responses of your variables that are printed out by the computer whenever you perform analyses using these variables.

> **Tip**
>
> Use value labels for specifying non-numeric responses and the measurement scale of numeric responses.

Each variable must have a name, which along with the variable type, should be indicated in your study manual. Most software programs accept variable names of up to eight letters/numbers/symbols. It is to your advantage to keep the names short because you will be typing them over and over again as you perform the statistical analyses.

Choose names for your variables that are descriptive and easy to remember. For example, when the name is within the length allowed by your program (e.g., age, race, income) use the full name. When possible, use familiar abbreviations (e.g., for the medicine hydrochlorothiazide the variable name should be HCTZ).

When you measure the same construct repeatedly, number the variables consecutively (e.g., for repeated measures of the CD4 lymphocyte count, name the variables CD4_1, CD4_2, etc.). By selecting descriptive names you will avoid having to constantly look back at your study manual to determine the name of a variable.

Most programs will also allow you to specify variable labels. Labels are descriptions of the variables that can be substantially longer than eight characters. They will be printed out whenever the program prints the variable name. For example, for a variable named madepbi6, you could specify the variable label: "maternal depression as measured by the Beck inventory at 6 months."

3.3.C Value labels

Value labels are descriptions of the different possible responses to your variables that are printed out by the computer whenever you perform analyses using these variables.

Value labels are particularly helpful for categorical variables such as race because the numbers associated with each response have no meaning. Value labels help you to remember whether "1" equals "African-American" or "Latino." They are also helpful for non-numeric responses such as "missing" or "non-applicable" (Section 3.3.D). For numeric responses on interval variables such as weight or blood pressure, the value label should indicate the scale or measurement (e.g., whether the variable weight was in kilograms or pounds).

3.3.D Alternative values

Besides the range of appropriate values, you must also consider how you will code alternative answers to your questions/variables such as:

- Don't know
- Can't remember
- Refused to answer
- Missing
- Other
- Does not apply

Although in your final analysis you may not distinguish these alternative answers it is important to retain the detail because each of these answers has a slightly different meaning. For example, if you ask people how many sexual partners they have had in the last year, prurient people may refuse to answer, whereas sexually adventuresome people may have had so many partners that they have lost count!

It is best to assign a symbol (e.g., " . ") rather than a number to alternative values. By using a symbol rather than a number such as "99", you will not inadvertently treat the missing value as if it were a real value (i.e., as if the patient's blood pressure really was 99 as opposed to the blood pressure value being missing).

> **Tip**
>
> To avoid mistakes, code alternative responses with symbols, not numbers.

3.4 How do I enter my data?

To enter your data into the computer you will need a database program. Although many statistical software programs (e.g., SAS, SPSS) allow you to enter data directly, generally they do not have the ease and flexibility of database programs. Therefore, you will want to enter your data into a database program and then "export" the data in a format that can be read by the statistical program (Figure 3.1).

If you are working with an established research group it is best to use whatever database program the others in your group are using. This way you can ask for help if you run into a problem. Commonly used commercially available database products include Access, DBASE Plus, FoxPro, and FileMaker Pro.

If you are starting out on your own, I would recommend one of two free data entry packages: EpiData or Epi Info. EpiData created by EpiData Association of Denmark (http://www.epidata.dk) is available free in over 10 languages, does not require a powerful computer, and exports data in formats that can be read by a large number of statistical and database programs.[38] Epi Info, also free

---

[38] For an excellent data management manual using EpiData see: Bennett, S., Myatt, M., Jolley, D., Radalowicz, A. *Data Management for Surveys and Trials* Denmark: EpiData Association, 2001, available free at http://www.gnu.org/copyleft/fdl.html.

(http://www.cdc.gov/epiinfo/), is easy to use and has the advantage of also per-forming basic statistical analyses.

The first step in entering data into a computer is to create the computer data entry screens. The goal of data entry screens is to minimize data entry errors. To accomplish this, design the screens to look like the paper questionnaires so that it is easy for the data entry staff to correctly enter the data.

A great advantage of modern database packages is that they allow you to program in range checks, skip logic, questions that must be answered, and con-sistency checks. For example, if you have specified that the acceptable range of systolic blood pressure is between 60 and 280 mmHg, the program will reject an entry below 60 or above 280. This is referred to as a range check. Range checks give you an opportunity to check whether the datum is accurate (e.g., perhaps 200 is being misread as 300).

Skip logic, also referred to as conditional jumps, means that if the subject answers a question in a particular way you skip certain questions (e.g., if the answer to question 6 is no, skip questions 7 through 10). Rather than have the interviewer or data entry person remember this, you can program your database to automatically skip certain questions depending on the answers to prior ques-tions that came before.

Must answer questions are questions that must be filled in with an answer other than missing. Date of birth is a question for which you would not expect to have any missing values.

Consistency checks require that answers to certain specified questions agree. For example, if you had a question about history of prior prostate can-cer, a response of yes would only be acceptable if the subject were male. Consistency checks are particularly useful with dates. For example, you might program in that the date of hospital discharge must occur after the date of hospital admission.

Although it takes a little extra time to program in these data checks, the time is well spent in terms of improving data quality.

If the data are being entered from a paper form it is best to have your data entered twice by two different data entry operators. The two versions are then compared using your data entry package. Any differences between the two are resolved by checking the original data. This is the only way you can find data entry errors that fall within normal values (e.g., one of the operators incor-rectly enters systolic blood pressure of 170 but the other operator enters it cor-rectly as 110). Having the same person enter the data twice is not as good because of the possibility of the operator making the same mistake twice (espe-cially if there is some ambiguity in the entry) but is better than having the data entered once.

Tip

Use range checks to identify values that are not plausible.

Tip

Use skip logic when answers to certain questions preclude answering subsequent questions.

Tip

It is best to have your data double entered by two different data entry operators.

3.5 How do I clean my data?

Cleaning data is like housecleaning. Few people enjoy it but it has got to be done! Fortunately, if you have incorporated range checks into your data entry processes, you should find data cleaning fairly easy!

The first step is to review the distribution of responses for each variable; the distribution of responses is referred to as the "frequencies" of your variables. The frequencies tell you how frequently each response to the variable occurs.

> **Tip**
>
> To clean your data run frequencies of all your variables.

Most database programs perform basic frequencies. If yours does not you will need to export your data to a statistical program (Section 3.9) prior to cleaning your data.

Review your frequencies for implausible values (these should be non-existent if you have set up your range checks correctly). Assess the amount of missing data you have on each question. Although some missing data are inevitable, variables with a lot of missing data may tip-off you off to a data entry problem. Ultimately, variables with a lot of missing data may need to be dropped from the analysis.

> **Tip**
>
> When cleaning your data look for implausible values, missing data, and sparse data.

Also, check the sample size of follow-up questions. For example, if 100 persons answered "no" to the question "Do you smoke?" then there should be 100 persons listed as "not applicable" for the question "How many cigarettes a day do you smoke?" If you find instead that there are 95 or 105 persons listed as non-applicable, figure out why by identifying the cases where the two questions do not agree and review the actual data.

Note variables with sparse data (i.e., variables with many values for which there are no or only a few subjects). These variables will generally need to be recoded (Section 3.6.A).

Do not wait until all your data is collected to clean it. Cleaning your data periodically during the data collection phase will enable you to spot problems that can be corrected before the study is over.

3.6 How do I recode a variable?

The two most common reasons for recoding data are to avoid sparse distributions and to reverse the direction of a variable.

3.6.A Sparse data

When you have variables with a sparse distribution of values (i.e., gaps where there are no or very few subjects with particular responses) it is often hard to see trends in your data. For example systolic blood pressure may vary in a sample from

60 to 240 mmHg. However, there may be very few subjects with systolic blood pressure <90 or >180 mmHg. Even between 90 and 180 mmHg there are 90 possible data points; therefore in a study of 200 people there will be few subjects at any one point.

In recoding interval variables such as blood pressure, effort should be made to retain the interval nature of the variable (i.e., maintain an equal interval between each of the values; Section 2.10). For example, systolic blood pressure can be recoded in tenths 60–69, 70–79, etc. If your data are very sparse, deciles may not be sufficient and you may need to recode the variable as <90, 90–109, 110–119, etc.[39]

At times you may wish to abandon the interval nature of a variable in order to categorize it into clinically meaningful groups. For example, in a study of mortality following a myocardial infarction, you might categorize systolic blood pressure as <90 (low blood pressure, suggestive of pump dysfunction), 90–139 (normal blood pressure), 140–159 (mildly elevated blood pressure), and 160 mmHg or higher (severely elevated blood pressure). Recoding the variable in this way changes it from an interval variable to an ordinal variable, thus limiting the types of statistical analyses that can performed using it. Yet such a change may be perfectly reasonable if it fits the goals of the study.

Sometimes interval variables are recoded into ordered categories such that each category has an equal or near equal number of subjects. For example, you might recode your variable into terciles (i.e., observations whose values are between 0% and 33% in group 1, 34% and 67% in group 2, etc.) or quartiles (i.e., observations whose values are between 0% and 24% in group 1, 25% and 49% in group 2, etc.). This strategy maximizes power by maintaining an equal distribution of values for the variable. It also prevents capitalizing on chance by recategorizing your variable using cut-offs chosen after reviewing the data. However, this type of recoding results in the loss of the interval nature of the variable.

Other times you will want to recode an interval variable by dichotomizing it. When dichotomizing variables it is best to use a clinically meaningful threshold (systolic blood pressure >140 mmHg; weight loss of 10 lb or more). For variables for which there is no such threshold (e.g., social support), variables can be dichotomized using median splits.

As implied by the name, a median split divides your sample into two parts: (1) all subjects with values less than the median and (2) all subjects with values greater than the mean. Subjects with values equal to the median can be placed in either group.

---

[39] Strictly speaking a variable that is recoded at the ends with < or > values is not an interval variable (because the categories with < or > values do not represent an equal interval to the other categories). But it is common to treat such variables as if they were interval.

The advantage of median splits as a method of dichotomizing a variable is that you have maximal power when your variable has an equal distribution of values. Of course, it you have a large number of subjects at the median, then splitting at the median will not result in an equal distribution of values in both groups. Also any time you dichotomize an interval variable there is a tremendous loss of information.

It is also important to check dichotomous, ordinal, and nominal variables for categories that have very few observations. No matter how important a category is to the theoretical basis of your study, if very few of your subjects fall into that category it is unlikely that you will have enough power to reveal important differences for that group.

For example, let us say you are performing a study of the impact of drug use on health care utilization among factory workers. A review of your dichotomous (yes/no) variables shows you that 70% of the workers report that they use alcohol, 20% report that they smoke cigarettes, and 0.8% report that they inject heroin. While heroin use may have a profound effect on health care use, it is unlikely that you will learn much about the impact of injecting heroin on health care use if <1% of respondents inject it. Therefore, the variable will need to be excluded from your study or you may be able to derive a new variable (Section 3.8) that includes it along with other substance use (e.g., any injection drug use or any illicit drug use).

In general, if you have powered your study to detect differences that assume relatively equal distributions of your independent variables, you are not at all likely to gain much information by looking at responses that are chosen by <5% of the sample.

Keep in mind as well that with dichotomous variables it does not matter which category has few observations. If 99.2% of your sample have recently injected heroin (as might be the case among participants in a heroin detoxification program) you also cannot study the impact of heroin use on health care utilization because everyone is a heroin user.

Uncommon responses can also be a problem with nominal variables. If you perform a survey of residents of Boston, Massachusetts, you may not have enough Mexican-Americans in your sample to learn about their health care experiences. On the other hand, if you survey residents of Phoenix, you may have enough Mexican-Americans but not enough African-Americans to understand their health care experience.

Categorizing uncommon responses as "other" is a handy way of reducing the number of categories without making subjects "missing" and thereby excluding them from the analysis. However, when you combine many different types of subjects together in an "other" category, you may obscure important differences: for

Tip

Responses chosen by <5% of the sample are unlikely to be informative unless you have a very large sample size.

Tip

Uncommon responses can be combined as "other."

Tip

When combining categories, be sure that you are not combining subjects with very different outcomes.

Table 3.1. Center for Epidemiologic Studies Depression Scale

	Rarely or none of the time (<1 day)	Some or little of the time (<1–2 days)	Occasionally or a moderate amount of the time (3–4 days)	Most or all of the time (5–7 days)
I was bothered by things that usually do not bother me. (CES-D1)*	0	1	2	3
I felt hopeful about the future. (CES-D2)*	0	1	2	3
I thought my life had been a failure. (CES-D3)*	0	1	2	3
I enjoyed life. (CES-D4)*	0	1	2	3

* Variable names are shown in parentheses.

example, some of the combined groups may have a high score and others a low score on the outcome. Also, the meaning of the other category can be hard to explain, if, for example, the "other" category has a significantly higher or lower rate of a particular disease.

3.6.B Reorienting variables

How a variable is oriented – whether a score of "1" means a better or worse performance than a score of "5" – makes no statistical difference. You will get the same statistical answer whether "1" is low and "5" is high or whether "1" is high and "5" is low (although the sign with certain statistics may be in the opposite direction).

However, the orientation of your variables matters if you wish to combine several variables together in one multi-item scale.[40] It would make no sense to summate 10 variables to obtain an overall score if a low number meant good performance on five of the questions and bad performance on the other five questions. Therefore, prior to combining questions into a scale, you must make sure all your variables are oriented in the same direction.

Let us use the 20-question Center for Epidemiologic Study of Depression Scale as an example.[41] For a variety of feelings and behaviors, subjects are asked: "Which statement best describes how often you felt or behaved this way – DURING THE PAST WEEK." The possible responses along with four representative items from the scale are shown in Table 3.1.

> **Tip**
>
> Prior to creating a scale, be sure that all the component variables are oriented in the same direction.

---

[40] For more on constructing scales, see: Katz, M.H. *Multivariable Analysis: A Practical Guide for Clinicians* (2nd edition). Cambridge: Cambridge University Press, 2005, 85–6.

[41] For more on scoring the CES-D and references on its use, see: www.huba.com/modules/ins_mod26score.htm

The final score is based on adding the responses of the 20 questions together. But it would make no sense to add the four questions in Table 3.1 together without first recoding two of them because a high score ("3") on the first and the third questions (CES-D1 and CES-D3) indicates depression while a low score ("0") on the second and fourth questions (CES-D2 and CES-D4) indicates depression. Thus, before adding them together you need to recode some of the items in the scale so that all the items are oriented in the same direction. Depending on the software package you are using the instructions will look something like this:

Recode CES-D2 $(0 = 3)(1 = 2)(2 = 1)(3 = 0)$

Recode CES-D4 $(0 = 3)(1 = 2)(2 = 1)(3 = 0)$

You may be asking yourself why not just orient all of the questions in the same direction in the first place? The answer is that you want to be sure that your participants are reading and considering each question carefully, not just circling one number assuming that all the questions ask essentially the same thing.

Even when you are not creating a scale, it may be desirable to orient all variables that measure a particular domain (such as mental health) in the same direction. For example, if you were looking at the association between alcohol consumption and mental health it would be easier to report the results if the anxiety and depression questions were both oriented in the same way (i.e., higher use of alcohol was associated with higher scores on the anxiety and depression scales).

3.6.C Final notes on recoding

> **Tip**
>
> Check the frequency of all recoded variables.

When you recode a variable, run a frequency (Section 4.3) on your new variable and a contingency table (Section 5.2) of your new variable versus your old variable. These analyses will enable you to be sure that the recoding was successful.

In recoding your variables, be sure you are not capitalizing on chance. For example, let us say that you note in your bivariate analysis (Chapter 4) that several categories of a nominal variable are high on a particular outcome. You therefore decide to group all the categories that are high on the outcome into one group and all the categories that are low on the outcome in the other group. You pat yourself on the back when you see the statistically significant result you have created! Not so fast! You have created this difference by capitalizing on chance: there will always be some categories that are higher than the mean, and some categories that are lower than the mean. If there was no a priori reason for combining these categories together you should not be grouping them together just to obtain a statistically significant result.

> **Tip**
>
> To avoid capitalizing on chance, do not recode categories based on their outcome.

3.7 How do I transform a variable?

Transforming a variable means changing the variable's scale of measurement. For example, to study the significance of CD4 lymphocyte counts (which range from 1 to $>1,000$) on prognosis of HIV-infected persons you may need to transform the variable CD4 lymphocyte count onto a logarithmic scale. The transformation of the variable CD4 would look something like this:

$$LOGCD4 = \log(CD4)$$

In other words you would create a new variable (LOGCD4) by taking the log of each subject's CD4 lymphocyte count (CD4). The most common reason for transforming a variable is so that it better fits the assumptions of the particular statistical model you wish use (Sections 5.4 and 6.5). Logarithm and square root are frequently used transformations.

3.8 When will I need to derive variables?

> The value of a derived variable depends on another variable(s) in your dataset.

A derived variable is a variable whose value depends on another variable(s) in your dataset. Derived variables are often necessary for determining intervals of time. For example, you may derive the variable "duration of time since prior hospitalization" by subtracting the date of study enrollment from the date of prior hospitalization.

Some important constructs are derived based on the answers to one or more questions. For example, the measure "pack years of smoking" is derived by multiplying the number of years smoked by the number of packs smoked per day for each subject.

After you have derived a variable, review the frequencies, just as you would for any variable, checking for implausible results. Be sure that any subject who is missing on any of the variables used to derive the new variable is assigned a missing value on the new derived variable. One exception to this rule: when the value of a variable derived from several variables does not change due to a missing value on one of the variables, you do not need to make the value for the derived variable missing for those cases. For example, if a subject answers "yes" to a question regarding cocaine use but leaves a question about heroin use blank, the derived value for the variable any illegal drug use can still be coded as "yes."

3.9 When should I export my data to a statistical program?

When to export your data from your database program to your statistical program (e.g., STATA, SAS) will depend on the ease with which your database program can do basic statistical analyses. For example, if you enter your data with Epi Info you may want to conduct all of the frequencies, *t*-tests, chi-squared tests, and other basic statistics with Epi-Info, and only export your data when you are ready to do multiple logistic or proportional hazards analysis. On the other hand, some data entry programs are not facile at performing even basic statistical analyses, and you will therefore export your data after running your frequencies and cleaning your data.

Univariate statistics

4.1 How should I describe my data?

The analysis of every study, whether a multimillion dollar multicenter randomized controlled trial of 100,000 patients or a descriptive study of one clinician's experience with 40 patients, should begin in the same way: with a review of the distribution of your variables. This is done using graphing techniques and univariate statistics.

You will sometimes see the term "univariate" used to refer to statistics that assess the relationship of two variables to each other. But since "uni" means one, it is preferable to reserve the term for analysis of a single variable and use bivariate analysis (Chapter 5) to refer to the relationship between two variables.

4.2 How should I describe my interval and ordinal variables?

Tip

Use histograms to describe interval and ordinal variables.

The first step in describing interval and ordinal variables is to visually review their distribution. This is done using a histogram.

Figure 4.1 shows a histogram of the estimated glomerular filtration rate (GFR) of 14,527 patients.[42]

Note that on a histogram each interval of a variable is represented as a rectangle sitting on a line (the line is usually horizontal, but histograms can also be shown on a vertical line); the line shows the range of possible values for the variable. The height of each rectangle indicates the frequency of the response (number of subjects or percentage of sample). Each rectangle is placed on the line at the center of the response (i.e., a rectangle representing 68–72 ml/min/1.73 m^2 of GFR would be positioned on the axis at 70 ml/min/1.73 m^2, the midpoint of the interval).

The width of the intervals of a histogram are chosen based on the density/ sparseness of the data. The interval should be as narrow as possible (so as not to

---

[42] Anavekar, N.S., McMurray, J.J.V., Velazquez, E.J., et al. Relation between renal dysfunction and cardiovascular outcomes after myocardial infarction. *New Engl. J. Med.* 2004; 351: 1285–95.

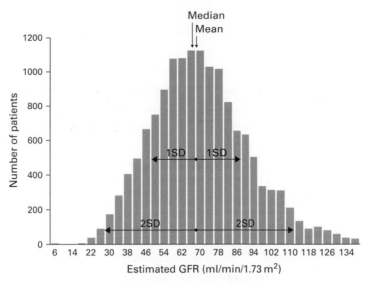

> The intervals of your histogram should be as narrow as possible while maintaining sufficient sample sizes in each interval.

blur trends in your data) while still maintaining sufficient subjects in each interval that you can see the patterns in your data. In general, larger sample sizes allow for much narrower intervals.

The arrow at the top of Figure 4.1 points to the mean value (GFR = 70 ml/min/1.73 m^2). The mean is the average value of the sample. It is computed as:

$$\text{average} = \text{mean} = \frac{\text{sum of values for all subjects}}{\text{number of subjects}}$$

> Normally distributed variables have a bell shape.

Note that the histogram for GFR values has a bell-shape: the largest number of patients has values near the mean of the GFR and there is an equal (symmetric) spread of values below and above (to the left and the right of) the mean. Variables that have a bell-shape histogram are said to have a normal distribution (also referred to as a Gaussian distribution).

> The "spread" of values around the mean is called the variance.

The "spread" of values around the mean is called the variance. In mathematical terms, the variance equals:

$$\text{variance} = \frac{(\text{average difference from the mean})^2}{(\text{sample size} - 1)}$$

We square the difference from the mean so that values that are an equal distance from the mean, whether above or below the mean, will contribute equally to the variance.

When the variance is small, the values for the subjects are close to the mean; when the variance is large, the values are far from the mean.

The spread around the mean can also be quantified using the standard deviation. It is calculated as the square root of the variance.

When a variable has a normal distribution, the standard deviation has a very useful property: approximately 68% of the observations fall within 1 standard deviation in each direction from the mean (total of 2 standard deviations), and about 95% of the observations fall within 2 standard deviations in each direction from the mean (total of 4 standard deviations).

> Variables that are normally distributed will have 68% of the observations within 1 standard deviation from the mean and 95% of the observations within 2 standard deviations from the mean.

In the case of the GFR illustrated in Figure 4.1, the standard deviation is $21 \, ml/min/1.73 \, m^2$. This means that we would expect about 68% of the patients to have a GFR between 49 $(70 - 21)$ and 91 $(70 + 21)$ and 95% of subjects would be expected to have a GFR between 28 $[70 - (2 \times 21)]$ and 112 $[70 + (2 \times 21)]$. From the horizontal arrows shown in Figure 4.1 you can see that this appears to be true.

Figure 4.2 shows the lipoprotein(a) levels of 2759 women.[43] Note that the distribution is not bell-shaped. The distribution of values is not symmetric around the mean. There are more subjects to the left of the mean (34) than to the right because the mean is being pulled to the right of the center of the distribution by the long tail.

Distributions such as the one shown in Figure 4.2 are referred to as skewed to the right (i.e., there is a long tail to the right of the peak). Variables can also be skewed to the left (i.e., a long tail to the left of the peak).

For skewed variables, report the median rather than the mean. The median is the observation at the 50%. If you order the observations from smallest to highest, the median is the value of the subject found at:

$$\frac{(N + 1)}{2}$$

The median (25 mg/dl) is a better description of the center of the distribution of lipoprotein(a) values than the mean (33.7 mg/dl) because it is unaffected by the extreme values at the tail of the distribution (Figure 4.2). With skewed distributions, 1 and 2 standard deviations in each direction will not necessarily encompass 68% and 95% of the sample, respectively.

---

[43] Shlipak, M.G., Simon, J.A., Vittinghoff, E., et al. Estrogen and progestin, lipoprotein(a), and the risk of recurrent coronary heart disease events after menopause. *J. Am. Med. Assoc.* 2000; 283: 1845–52.

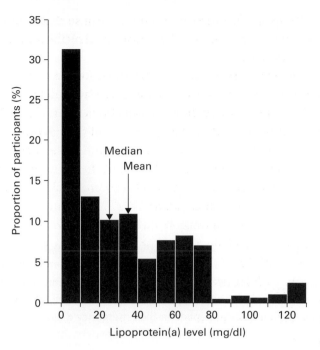

> Your distribution is likely
> skewed if the mean and
> the median substantially
> differ from one another
> or if the standard
> deviation is as big or
> bigger than the mean.

Besides the appearance of the histogram, a tip off that you have a skewed distribution is if the mean and the median are substantially different from one another. In this regard note that the mean and median are almost identical for Figure 4.1 (70 and 69 ml/min/1.73 m^2) but not for Figure 4.2. Another indication of a skewed distribution is if the standard deviation is as big or bigger than the mean. For example, the standard deviation for the lipoprotein(a) levels shown in Figure 4.2 is the same size (33 mg/dl) as the mean.

As the standard deviation of a non-normally distributed variable is not a valid indicator of the distribution, the distribution of a non-normally distributed variable should be reported using the 25% and 75%, often referred to as the interquartile range. It indicates the values for the central half of your sample. As a study may have both normally and non-normally distributed variables, it is often best to report all your interval variables using the median and the interquartile range.

A nice way to illustrate the median and the interquartile range is to use box plots. For example, Maisel and colleagues used a box plot to illustrate the B-type natriuretic peptide levels of 744 patients with dyspnea due to congestive heart

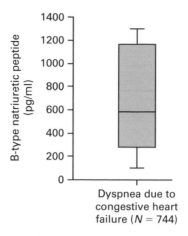

Figure 4.3

Box plot of B-type natriuretic peptide levels of 744 patients with dyspnea due to congestive heart failure. The box shows the interquartile range, the T-bars represent the highest and lowest values, and the horizontal line in the middle is the median. Reproduced with permission from Maisel, A.S., et al. Rapid measurement of B-type natriuretic peptide in the emergency diagnosis of heart failure. *New Engl. J. Med.* 2002; 347: 161–7. Copyright 2000 Massachusetts Medical Society. All rights reserved.

Tip

Use the median and the 25% and 75% (interquartile range) to describe non-normally distributed variables.

Definition

The mode is the most frequently occurring response.

failure (Figure 4.3) seen in the emergency department.[44] The box shows the interquartile range and the T-bars represent the highest and lowest values (the range). The horizontal line in the middle is the median. Sometimes box plots will also include a horizontal line showing the mean. Outlier points (an observation point that markedly deviates from the other observations in the sample) may be shown above or below the T-bars.

Another descriptor of a variable's distribution is the mode. The mode is the most frequently occurring response. With a normally distributed variable, the mode will be near the mean and the median.

With a bimodal distribution (another type of non-normal distribution) the most common responses are seen at two points that are separate from one another (technically speaking, a distribution cannot have two modes, unless the humps are exactly equal, but the term bimodal is used nonetheless).

For example, Pia and colleagues found that the results of tuberculin skin testing in 720 health care workers had a bimodal distribution (Figure 4.4).[45] The first peak occurred near 0 mm and the second peak occurred near 15 mm.

---

[44] Maisel, A.S., Krishnaswamy, P., Nowak, R.M. Rapid measurement of B-type natriuretic peptide in the emergency diagnosis of heart failure. *New Engl. J. Med.* 2002; 347: 161–7.

[45] Pai, M., Gokhale, K., Joshi, R., et al. *Mycobacterium tuberculosis* infection in health care workers in rural India. *J. Am. Med. Assoc.* 2005; 293: 2746–55.

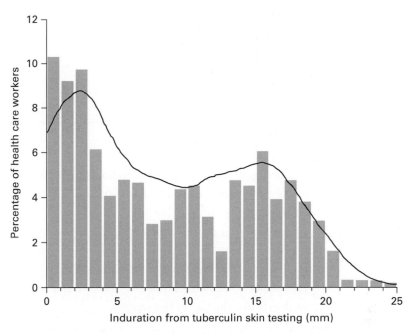

Figure 4.4   A bimodal distribution of skin induration from tuberculin skin testing among 720 health care workers. The overlaid curve is a smoothed version of the histogram. Adapted with permission from Pai, M., et al. *Mycobacterium tuberculosis* infection in health care workers in rural India. *J. Am. Med. Assoc.* 2005; 293: 2746–55. Copyright 2005 American Medical Association. All rights reserved.

> A variable with a normal distribution will graph as a straight line on a normal probability plot.

Another way of telling whether a variable has a normal distribution is to graph your data using a normal probability plot (many statistical programs will print this out for you). If your data are normally distributed, the values will appear as a straight line.[46] You can also review the statistics skewness and kurtosis; when they are high the variable is not normally distributed.

4.3 How should I describe my dichotomous variables?

Dichotomous variables are described by showing the frequencies of each response to the variable. Frequency tables show you the absolute number and the relative frequencies (percentage) of each response to a specific variable (Table 4.1).

Remember that the percentage is simply the proportion multiplied by 100. As they are mathematically interchangeable I will use percentage and proportion interchangeably throughout the book.

---

[46] Vittinghoff, E., Glidden, D.V., Shiboski, S.C., McCulloch, C.E. *Regression Methods in Biostatistics.* New York: Springer, 2005, p. 13.

Table 4.1. Simple frequency table

Hypertension	Number	Percent	Cumulative percent
0 "No"	70	70	70
1 "Yes"	30	30	100
Total	100	100	

Mean = 0.3.

It is best to use value labels with dichotomous variables (Section 3.3.C); otherwise the computer will just print out "0" and "1" and you may become confused as to whether 1 is "Yes" or "No".

In the case of a dichotomous variable, if you have coded it as "0" when the condition is absent and "1" when the condition is present, then the mean of the variable equals the prevalence of the condition.

Prevalence equals the number of cases who have a condition at a moment in time divided by the size of the sample:[47]

$$\text{prevalence} = \frac{\text{number of cases at a particular moment}}{\text{size of sample}}$$

> **Tip**
>
> The percentage is the proportion multiplied by 100.

> **Tip**
>
> Code dichotomous variable as "0" (condition absent) and "1" (condition present) so that the mean will equal the prevalence of the condition.

> **Definition**
>
> Confidence intervals quantify the uncertainty of a point estimate.

When reporting the prevalence of a disease (or any proportion) it is important to report the confidence intervals for the proportion. Confidence intervals (CI) are a method of quantifying the uncertainty around a particular point estimate, such as a proportion.[48]

Intuitively, it makes sense that if you sample a population repeatedly you will not find exactly the same percentage of persons with a particular condition. Some samples will yield a higher frequency and others will yield a lower frequency.

The 95% confidence intervals (the ones most commonly used) tell you that for 95% of the repeated samples the confidence interval will include the true value. Unfortunately, you cannot tell whether yours is one of the 95% or the other 5%! More generally, the confidence interval is the range of "answers" that are compatible with your data, taking into account sampling error.

In reporting the prevalence of a disease, the usual format is: the prevalence of disease is X% (95% CI = X% to X%).

---

[47] For more on prevalence see: Fletcher, R.H., Fletcher, S.W., Wagner, EH. *Clinical Epidemiology: The Essential* (3rd edition). pp. 76–7, 79–80; Hennekens, C.H., Buring, J.E. *Epidemiology in Medicine.* Boston: Little, Brown and Company, 1987, pp. 57, 63–4.

[48] Confidence intervals can be constructed for a variety of point estimates including the mean of an interval variable. However, I didn't raise the issue of confidence intervals earlier because most investigators report the standard deviation of a mean rather than the confidence intervals of the mean, although they convey different information and they are both relevant.

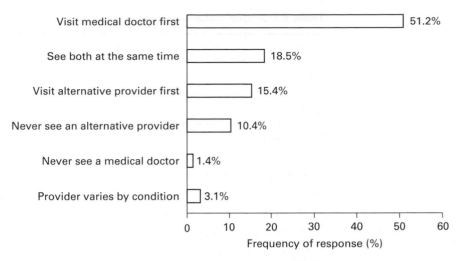

Figure 4.5   Bar graph shows sequence of seeking care from medical doctors and alternative medical providers (*n* = 411). Reprinted with permission from Eisenberg, D.M., et al. Perceptions about complimentary therapies relative to conventional therapies among adults who use both: results from a national survey. *Ann. Intern. Med.* 2001; 135: 344–51.

Although it is standard to report the 95% confidence intervals, there is nothing magical about the probability of 95%. If you want a higher probability that repeated samples would yield confidence intervals that include the true value you can report 99% confidence intervals. Conversely, if you are willing to tolerate a lower percentage of samples yielding confidence intervals that include the true value you can report 90% confidence intervals.

4.4 How should I describe my nominal variables?

Nominal variables are described using bar graphs and frequency tables. Bar graphs are similar to histograms: each response is represented by a rectangle. The height of the rectangle (or length when oriented vertically like Figure 4.5) equals the number or frequency of response. In contrast to histograms, the rectangles are not contiguous but are spaced evenly apart and the order of the rectangles makes no difference.

For example, Eisenberg et al. asked 411 subjects who said they saw both a medical doctor and an alternative medical provider about the sequence in which they saw them.[49] The results are shown in Figure 4.5 and Table 4.2. Note

---

[49] Eisenberg, D.M., Kessler, R.C., Van Rompay, M.I., et al. Perceptions about complimentary therapies relative to conventional therapies among adults who use both: results from a national survey. *Ann. Intern. Med.* 2001; 135: 344–51.

Table 4.2. Frequency table showing sequence of seeking care from medical doctors and alternative providers

	Number	Percent	Cumulative percent
1. Visit medical doctor first	210	51.2	51.2
2. See both at the same time	76	18.5	69.7
3. Visit alternative provider first	63	15.4	85.1
4. Never see an alternative provider	43	10.4	95.5
5. Never see a medical doctor	6	1.4	96.9
6. Provider varies by condition	13	3.1	100.0
Total	411	100.0	

Mean = 2.02 (nonsense!)

Data from Eisenberg, D.M., et al. Perceptions about complimentary therapies relative to conventional therapies among adults who use both: results from a national survey. *Ann. Intern. Med.* 2001; 135: 344–51.

that for Figure 4.5, you could put the rectangles in any order without changing the meaning of the graph. This is not true of the histograms shown in Figures 4.1, 4.2, and 4.4.

The bar graph gives the reader a better sense of the data than the frequency table, but the frequency table can be more helpful for the investigator for cleaning and recoding data, and pursuing further analyses.

The cumulative percentage from the frequency table shows you the groups to which the majority of your subjects belong. In this case over two-thirds of the sample visit a medical doctor first or at the same time as an alternative provider.

Even though it is nonsense, I have put the mean at the bottom of Table 4.2 to remind you that even if a variable is nominal, a statistical program may compute a mean for the variable. If you have assigned numbers to each category (which is the usual practice), the computer has no way of knowing that the variable is nominal, and will compute statistics as if the variable is interval.

4.5 How should I describe ordinal variables?

Ordinal variables are generally described in the same way as nominal variables, using bar graphs and frequency tables. The only difference is that the categories should be shown in numeric order.

4.6 How should I describe events that occur over time?

Thus far, we have considered in this chapter how to describe events or conditions that are observed at a particular point in time (e.g., estimated GFR, presence of hypertension).

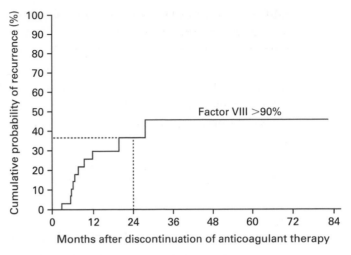

Number of patients at risk

| Factor VIII > 90% | 35 | 19 | 7 | 4 | 4 | 2 | 1 | 0 |

Figure 4.6   Kaplan–Meier curve describing the likelihood of a recurrent thromboembolism among patients with elevated Factor VIII levels over a 6-year period. Adapted with permission from Kyrle, P.A., et al. High plasma levels of factor VII and the risk of recurrent venous thromboembolism. *New Engl. J. Med.* 2000; 343: 457–62. Copyright 2000 Massachusetts Medical Society. All rights reserved.

However, often in clinical medicine we are interested in events (e.g., cancer occurrence, death) that occur over time. There are two major methods for describing time to outcome: survival curves and incidence rates.

4.6.A Survival curves

Survival curves describe the proportion of persons experiencing an event over a period of time (e.g., death over a 5-year period). They can also be set up to assess the proportion of persons not experiencing an outcome over a period of time (e.g., disease-free or remission times).

> Kaplan–Meier curves are used to describe the proportion of subjects experiencing an outcome over time.

The Kaplan–Meier method (also called the product-limit method) is the most common method for calculating a survival curve. For example, Figure 4.6 shows a Kaplan–Meier curve describing the likelihood of a recurrent thromboembolism among patients with elevated Factor VIII levels over a 6-year period.[50] Patients with elevated Factor VIII levels are known to be more likely to have thromboembolism.

---

[50] Kyrle, P.A., Minar, E., Hirschl, M., et al. High plasma levels of factor VII and the risk of recurrent venous thromboembolism. *New Engl. J. Med.* 2000; 343: 457–62.

By convention the x-axis of the Kaplan–Meier curve represents time since the start of the study. In the case of this study, time (x-axis) starts at the time that patients discontinued anticoagulant therapy for their first embolism.

The y-axis represents the proportion of participants who have (or have not) experienced the outcome at each point in time. Depending upon the outcome you are studying, the y-axis may be labeled cumulative probability, probability of survival, proportional mortality, etc. In epidemiologic terms it is known as the incidence proportion or the cumulative incidence rate (although it is a proportion not a rate).

In the case of Figure 4.6 the y-axis equals the cumulative probability of a recurrent thromboembolism. Therefore at time 0, no one has had a thromboembolism. It would be equally valid to have the y-axis represent the proportion of persons who were recurrence-free, in which case at time 0 the graph would show 100% without recurrence. The way you set up the graph makes no statistical difference.

Kaplan–Meier graphs look like a staircase. Each step represents one or more subjects who have experienced an outcome. When more than one subject experiences an outcome, the step is larger. The step size also increases as the study progresses because there are fewer persons at risk.

You can tell the number of persons at risk based on the legend below the curve. Every Kaplan–Meier curve should have a legend like Figure 4.6. All patients are at risk at the start of the study. They cease to be at risk when they experience the outcome or when there is no further follow-up information (see discussion of censoring below). It is important to know the number of persons at risk at each time point because when the number at risk is small, you cannot have as much confidence in the results at that point in time. For this reason, some researchers will truncate their curves so as not to suggest that there is accurate data beyond a certain point in time. In the case of this study, it would have been reasonable to truncate the curve at 2–3 years, when the number of persons at risk dropped below six or seven.

The point at which 50% of the subjects have experienced the outcome is referred to as the median survival time. According to Figure 4.6 what is the median time to recurrence of thromboembolism? Trick question. You cannot determine it because half the subjects have not experienced the outcome (have not had a recurrence).

Mean time to outcome can be calculated for Kaplan–Meier curves but is not generally reported because it is often skewed by a few subjects with very long times to outcome.

However, at any point in time you can determine the proportion of persons who have already experienced the outcome. I have drawn dotted lines on Figure 5.6 to

Below every Kaplan–Meier curve there should be a legend showing the number of persons at risk.

Median survival time is the point at which 50% of the subjects have experienced the outcome.

Tip

Median survival time cannot be calculated unless half the subjects have experienced the outcome.

show you how to determine the proportion of the sample that have had a recurrent thromboembolism by 2 years (37%).

You might ask at this point: Why do I need to draw Kaplan–Meier curves to determine the proportion of persons who have experienced the outcome by a particular point in time? Why can't I simply divide the number of persons who have experienced the outcome by the sample size? The answer is that you could if you have full follow-up for all subjects. Unfortunately, this is rarely the case with longitudinal studies. Subjects move, refuse further evaluation, or are lost to follow-up for unknown reasons. Subjects develop outcomes that preclude the outcome that is being studied (e.g., a subject in an AIDS drug trial may die of a heroin overdose). Subjects are withdrawn because they experience events that preclude them from continuing in the study (e.g., a patient may develop renal failure and therefore be unable to take the study medication).

Kaplan–Meier curves enable us to include subjects with differing lengths of follow-up by *censoring* subjects who do not experience the outcome of interest at the time they leave the analysis. Censoring is a major element of all types of survival analyses. Subjects are considered censored if they are lost to follow-up, experience an outcome that precludes the outcome of interest, or are withdrawn. Also subjects who do not experience the outcome by the end of the study are censored at the end of the study.

> Survival analyses assume that censoring occurs randomly, independent of outcome.

Survival analyses assume that censored persons, if they had not been censored, would have had the same course as those not censored. Another way of saying this is that the censoring occurs randomly, independent of outcome. This assumption allows censored persons to be included in the analysis until they leave the study.

This is a very problematic assumption because it is impossible to prove that censored observations have the same experience as those uncensored. Indeed, several studies have found that subjects who dropout are different than subjects who remain in the trial.

What should you do? For starters, censored observations are less likely to be a problem if few subjects are censored prior to the end of the study. If you have more than a few censored observations (say more than 5%) prior to the end of the study, the readers (and the reviewers) will justifiably worry whether the censoring assumption is reasonable.

> To assess the censoring assumption compare the characteristics of censored subjects to uncensored subjects.

Second, you can test the validity of the censoring assumption by comparing the baseline characteristics of subjects who dropped out to those who remained in the study. If you have collected data on important parameters during the study (but prior to dropouts), compare persons who dropped out and those who stayed in the study on these characteristics as well. If the subjects censored prior to the end of the study are similar to those who remained in the study, readers are likely to be reassured.

Another method to assess whether censoring occurred randomly in your study is to graphically compare the patterns of censored observations. If the patterns are different (e.g., a lot of the censored observations occurred early in one arm of the study and late in the other) then the censoring assumption may not be valid.[51]

Another important assumption of Kaplan–Meier curves is that if you have enrolled subjects over a period of time, there are no major temporal trends. Otherwise, the experience of subjects enrolled late may be different than that of subjects enrolled early. The Kaplan-Meier curve will then be affected by the proportion of subjects enrolled at each time period rather than the underlying experience of the sample.

4.6.B Incidence rates

A second method of describing time to outcome is to calculate incidence rate (also known as the incidence density) by pooling person observation time. The incidence rate is calculated as:

$$\text{incidence rate} = \frac{\text{number of new cases of disease}}{\text{number of persons at risk per unit time}}$$

Unlike the incidence proportion which can vary between 0 and 1 (Section 4.6.A), the incidence rate varies from 0 to infinity.

Soteriades and colleagues calculated the incidence rate of syncope among the participants in the Framingham Heart Study and the Framingham Offspring Study[52] (Section 2.6.B). They followed 7814 participants for an average of 17.0 years. During 133,164 person-years of follow-up, 822 participants developed syncope. Therefore the incidence rate is:

$$\text{incidence rate} = \frac{822}{133,164 \text{ person-years}} = 0.0062 \text{ per person-year}$$
$$= 6.2 \text{ per thousand person-years}$$

The person-years of follow-up is based on adding the amount of at-risk time each participant contributes to the analysis. If a participant drops-out of the study, or develops an outcome that precludes development of the outcome under study (e.g., death in a study of the incidence of stroke), or is withdrawn

---

[51] For more on computation of Kaplan–Meier curves with censored observations, and how to test the assumptions underlying censoring, see Katz, M.H. *Multivariable Analysis: A Practical Guide for Clinicians* (2nd edition). Cambridge: Cambridge University Press, 2005, pp. 29–32, 56–67.

[52] Soteriades, E.S., Evans, J.C., Larson, M.G., et al. Incidence and prognosis of syncope. *New Engl. J. Med.* 2002; 347: 878–85.

from a study (may occur if the subject experiences a side effect to a drug being tested), the participant ceases to contribute follow-up time. Also, once a participant has a syncopal episode they cease to contribute follow-up time.

The assumptions underlying calculation of incidence rates are similar to those underlying Kaplan–Meier curves. Specifically, for incidence rates to be valid the likelihood of outcome for subjects that dropout, develop an alternative outcome, or are withdrawn must be the same as that for subjects who continue in the study. There must also be no temporal changes during the period being summarized by a single rate.

As they convey similar types of information, longitudinal studies may report Kaplan–Meier curves, incident rates, or both. When you are interested in seeing how the occurrence of events changes over time use Kaplan–Meier curves rather than incident rates. The reason is that for incident rates to be valid the rate of events should be approximately constant over the time interval being studied.[53]

---

[53] The assumption of constant risk within an interval is also true of Kaplan–Meier curves. However, an interval in a Kaplan–Meier curve is defined by the occurrence of an outcome; therefore, these intervals are very short thereby fulfilling the assumption of constant risk throughout the interval. For more on the similarities and differences of Kaplan–Meier and incident risk for longitudinal data see Rosner, B. *Fundamentals of Biostatistics* (5th edition). Pacific Grove, CA: Duxbury, 2000, pp. 677–738; Kahn, H.A. Sempos, C.T. *Statistical Methods in Epidemiology*. Oxford: Oxford University Press, 1989, pp. 168–224.

Bivariate statistics

5.1 How do I assess an association between two variables?

Choose the bivariate statistic based on the type of risk factor and outcome variable you have.

There are more than 10 commonly used statistics for demonstrating an association between two variables. But have no fear! Choosing the correct one is not difficult. You choose the bivariate statistic based on: (1) the type of risk factor and outcome variable you have; and (2) whether the data are unpaired or paired (repeated observations or matched data). Bivariate statistics for unpaired data are shown in Table 5.1.[54] Bivariate statistics for repeated observations and matched data are shown in Tables 5.22 and 5.28 and discussed in Sections 5.10 and 5.11.

5.2 How do I assess an association between two dichotomous variables (comparison of proportions)?

The most commonly used tests for the association between two dichotomous variables with unpaired data are the chi-squared test[55] and Fisher's exact test.[56]

It is easiest to follow these tests if you think of them in terms of a two-by-two contingency table (also referred to as a cross tabulation table) as shown in Table 5.2. (It is called a two-by-two table because it has two rows and two columns.)

In a two-by-two table, each subject will fall into one of the four cells – labeled a, b, c, d – depending on that subject's values on the risk factor and the outcome. The column totals ($a + c$ and $b + d$) and the row totals ($a + b$ and $c + d$) are referred to as marginal totals.

---

[54] For more detailed explanations of the statistics covered in this chapter, see Glantz, S.A. *Primer of Biostatistics* (5th edition). New York: McGraw-Hill, 2002.

[55] Until recently, I referred to this test, like most textbooks, as chi-square (without the *d*). Although this is common usage, the name of the test is the Greek letter chi-squared (χ^2). Just as we would say that 2^2 is two-squared, not two-square, χ^2 is chi-squared, not chi-square.

[56] For a more detailed discussion of these two and other statistics for comparing two dichotomous variables see: Fleiss, J.L., Levin, B., Paik, M.C. *Statistical Methods for Rates and Proportions* (3rd edition). Hoboken, New Jersey: Wiley & Sons, 2003.

Table 5.1. Statistics for assessing an association between two variables, unpaired data

Risk factor (independent variable, exposure, group assignment)	Outcome (dependent variable)					
	Dichotomous	Nominal	Interval, normal distribution	Interval non-normal	Ordinal	Time to event, censored data
Dichotomous	Chi-squared, Fisher's exact test, risk ratio, odds ratio	Chi-squared	t-test	Mann-Whitney test	Chi-squared for trend, Mann-Whitney test	Log-rank, Wilcoxon, rate ratio
Nominal	Chi-squared, exact test	Chi-squared	ANOVA	Kruskal–Wallis test	Kruskal–Wallis test	Log-rank, Wilcoxon
Interval, normal distribution	t-test	ANOVA	Linear regression, Pearson's correlation coefficient	Spearman's rank correlation coefficient	Spearman's rank correlation coefficient	–
Interval, non-normal	Mann-Whitney test	Kruskal–Wallis test	Spearman's rank correlation coefficient	Spearman's rank correlation coefficient	Spearman's rank correlation coefficient	–
Ordinal	Chi-squared for trend, Mann-Whitney test	Kruskal–Wallis test	Spearman's rank correlation coefficient	Spearman's rank correlation coefficient	Spearman's rank correlation coefficient	–

Table 5.2. Two-by-two contingency table

Risk factor (independent variable, exposure, group assignment)	Outcome (dependent variable, case and control)		Total
	Yes	No	
Yes	a	b	$a + b$
No	c	d	$c + d$
Total	$a + c$	$b + d$	

Although it makes no statistical difference, the convention is to put the risk factor (also referred to as: independent variable, exposure, or group assignment[57]) as the row and the outcome (also referred to as: dependent variable) as the column. Typically, the risk factor is present in the top row and absent in the bottom row, and the outcome is present in the left column and absent in the right column.

In parentheses in Tables 5.1 and 5.2, I have included the synonyms for the risk factor and outcome to remind you that the underlying statistics are the same regardless of what names are used. The names are generally chosen based on the type of study being performed: cohort (risk factor and outcome), case–control (exposure and case and control), and randomized controlled trials (group assignment and outcome).

Keep in mind that when you test the association of two dichotomous variables, what you are really doing is comparing two proportions. Each row produces a proportion: the proportion of subjects with the risk factor who experience the outcome $[a/(a + b)]$ and the proportion of subjects without the risk factor who experience the outcome $[c/(c + d)]$.

The chi-squared statistic tests the association between two dichotomous variables by comparing the number of subjects who would be expected to be in each cell of the cross-tabulation table, assuming no association between the two variables, to the observed number of subjects in each cell.

When the observed number of subjects in each cell is very different than the expected number (i.e., when the proportion of subjects experiencing the outcome differs between the two groups) there is an association between the two variables. This is reflected in a large chi-squared and a small P-value. If the P-value is below the conventionally used threshold of $P < 0.05$, we say that the result is statistically significant, meaning that the observed association is unlikely to have occurred by chance.

> **Tip**
>
> Bivariate tests of dichotomous variables are comparisons of proportions.

> **Definition**
>
> Chi-squared compares the expected cell number to the observed cell number.

---

[57] A fourth term commonly used interchangeably with the other three is predictor. However, I prefer to restrict the term prediction to situations where we are trying to predict the outcomes for particular subjects.

Table 5.3. Marginal totals for association between diabetes and death

Diabetes	Death		Total
	Yes	No	
Yes			726 (14.72)
No			4206 (85.28)
Total	205	4727	4932 (100)

Values are represented as n (%).

Table 5.4. Association between diabetes and death assuming the null hypothesis is true

Diabetes	Death		Total
	Yes	No	
Yes	30 (14.7)	696 (14.7)	726 (14.72)
No	175 (85.3)	4031 (85.3)	4206 (85.28)
Total	205	4727	4932 (100)

Values are represented as n (%).

To illustrate how the chi-squared test works let's examine data on the impact of diabetes on death. Bobrie and colleagues[58] followed 4932 persons with hypertension, of whom 205 (4%) died during the 3-year follow-up period.

Table 5.3 shows the marginal totals for each column and row from the study. You can see that at baseline 726 (14.72%) persons had diabetes and 4206 (85.28%) did not have diabetes.[59]

Is the presence of diabetes associated with death? You cannot tell from the marginal totals. You need to see the empty cells filled in. But before I fill them in with the actual data, let us fill them in assuming that the null hypothesis is true: that diabetes is not associated with death.

If diabetes were not associated with death then we would expect that there would be no difference between the percentage of diabetics who died and the percentage of diabetics who were still alive at the end of the follow-up period. We know from Table 5.4 that diabetics represent 14.72% of the sample. Therefore, if

[58] Bobrie, G., Chatellier, G., Genes, N., et al. Cardiovascular prognosis of "masked hypertension" detected by blood pressure self-measurement in elderly treated hypertensive patients. *J. Am. Med. Assoc.* 2004; 291: 1342–9.

[59] Typically, I would not show more than one decimal place for a percentage because it implies a greater level of precision than these numbers have. However, if I round off the percentages the multiplication below will result in the numbers not adding up correctly across the rows.

Table 5.5. Actual data showing association between diabetes and death

Diabetes	Death		Total
	Yes	No	
Yes	47 (22.9)	679 (14.4)	726 (14.7)
No	158 (77.1)	4048 (85.6)	4206 (85.3)
Total	205	4727	4932 (100)

Values are represented as n (%).
$\chi^2 = 11.48$; $P = 0.0007$.
Data from Bobrie, G., et al. Cardiovascular prognosis of "masked hypertension" detected by blood pressure self-management in elderly treated hypertensive patients. *J. Am. Med. Assoc.* 2004; 291: 1342–9.

Table 5.6. Determination of degrees of freedom for a two-by-two table

Diabetes	Death		Total
	Yes	No	
Yes	47		726 (14.72)
No			4206 (85.28)
Total	205	4727	4932 (100)

Values are represented as n (%).

the null hypothesis were true than we would expect that diabetics would represent 14.72% of the deaths and 14.72% of the persons still alive. Similarly, we would expect that persons without diabetes would represent 85.28% of the deaths and 85.28% of the non-deaths.

To determine the number of subjects in each cell perform multiplication as shown below:

Death among persons with diabetes $= 0.1472 \times 205 = 30$
No death among persons with diabetes $= 0.1472 \times 4727 = 696$
Death among persons without diabetes $= 0.8528 \times 205 = 175$
No death among persons without diabetes $= 0.8528 \times 4727 = 4031$

We can now fill in the two-by-two table (Table 5.4) assuming the null hypothesis is true.

In Table 5.5, I have placed the actual data on the relationship between diabetes and death.

Comparing Tables 5.4 and 5.5 you can see that the actual results differ substantially from what was expected if the null hypothesis were true. Forty-seven

Definition

The degrees of freedom are the number of independent units of information used to calculate a particular statistic.

diabetics died although we anticipated only 30 would have died. Among persons without diabetes 679 died but we had anticipated 696 would have died. This is why the chi-squared is large.

To determine the *P*-value from the chi-squared test you have to know the degrees of freedom. The degrees of freedom are the number of independent units of information used to calculate a particular statistic.

Although this may sound complicated, Table 5.6 illustrates how easy this is to determine for a two-by-two table. I have filled in cell "*a*". From this one cell there is only one way you can fill in the other three cells of the table (e.g., $b = 726 - 47 = 679, d = 4727 - 679 = 4048$, etc.). This means that a two-by-two table has only one degree of freedom.

Knowing the chi-squared value and the degrees of freedom you can determine the *P*-value from the tables that used to be at the back of every statistic book. In this computer age, it is rare to look up the probability of a test result using a table. This is done by the computer (and therefore I have not placed any statistical tables at the back of this book!). You will see the number of degrees of freedom often printed out next to your analysis; it is helpful to know what it means.

To obtain a valid chi-squared test, the *expected* number of subjects per cell must be at least 5. I have italicized the word expected to remind you that it is not the observed number of subjects per cell that determines whether the chi-squared is valid. This means that with small sample sizes (e.g., <50) you need to determine the expected number of subjects per cell before using the chi-squared test. This would be tedious to do by hand. Fortunately, most computer programs will tell you automatically if the expected number of subjects is <5 in any cell of the table.

For example, Villar and colleagues investigated the cause of a botulism outbreak among bus drivers in Argentina.[60] One of the foods they investigated is *matambre*, a traditional meat dish of Argentina that is cooked at temperatures too low to kill *Clostridium botulinum* spores.

As with the diabetes example, let us start with the marginal totals (Table 5.7).

To determine the number of subjects expected in each cell, we fill in the cells of the table assuming that the null hypothesis is true.

If eating *matambre* were not associated with botulism we would expect that bus drivers who ate *matambre* would represent an equal proportion of cases and non-cases of botulism. We know from the marginal totals in Table 5.7 that 52% of the drivers ate *matambre* and 48% did not. Therefore, if the null hypothesis were true than we would expect that 52% of the botulism cases and 52% of the non-cases ate *matambre*.

---

[60] Villar, R.G., Shapiro, R.L., Busto, S. Outbreak of Type A botulism and development of a botulism surveillance and antitoxin release system in Argentina. *J. Am. Med. Assoc.* 1999; 281: 1334–8, 1340.

Table 5.7. Marginal totals for association between consumption of matambre and botulism

| Ate *matambre* | Botulism | | |
	Yes	No	Total
Yes			11 (52)
No			10 (48)
Total	9	12	21 (100)

Values are represented as *n* (%).

To determine the expected number of subjects in each cell perform multiplication as shown below:

Botulism among eaters of *matambre* $= 0.52 \times 9 = 5$

No botulism among eaters of *matambre* $= 0.52 \times 12 = 6$

Botulism among non-eaters of *matambre* $= 0.48 \times 9 = 4$

No botulism among non-eaters of *matambre* $= 0.48 \times 12 = 6$

As the bolded cell is expected to have fewer than 5 subjects it would not be valid to use the chi-squared test. Instead, use Fisher's exact test to assess the association between two dichotomous variables when the expected cell frequency is <5 subjects. It is never wrong to use the Fisher's exact test instead of chi-squared. The major reason we traditionally used chi-squared test, where applicable, rather than the Fisher's exact test is that the latter is computationally much more difficult. However, with the increased speed of modern computers this has become much less of an issue.

Fisher's exact test determines the probability of obtaining a particular pattern of data given all possible arrangements of the observations. Fisher's exact test can be computed assuming one or two tails; you will almost always want to use the two-tailed test (Section 2.8).

Table 5.8 shows the actual data on the association between consumption of *matambre* and botulism. You can see that there is a very strong relationship between eating *matambre* and developing botulism. The probability of getting such an association by chance is very small, reflected in the significant *P*-value for the Fisher's exact test.

A limitation of both the chi-squared and Fisher's exact test is that they do not measure the strength of the association between the risk factor and the outcome. (If you were thinking that a small *P*-value told you that it was a strong relationship remember the example of the tossed coin (Section 1.1)). *P*-values only tell you the probability that the observed association could have occurred by chance if there were no true association between eating *matambre* and botulism. With large sample sizes even small differences may be statistically significant.

Table 5.8. Actual data showing association between consumption of matambre and botulism

| | Botulism | | |
Ate *matambre*	Yes	No	Total
Yes	9 (82)	2 (18)	11 (52)
No	0 (0)	10 (100)	10 (48)
Total	9	12	21 (100)

Values are represented as n (%).
Fisher's exact test (two-tailed) = 0.0002.
Data from Villar, R.G., et al. Outbreak of Type A botulism and development of a botulism surveillance and antitoxin release system in Argentina. *J. Am. Med. Assoc.* 1999; 281: 1334–8, 1340.

Definition

The risk ratio is the ratio of the probability of occurrence in one group to the probability of occurrence in the other group.

Two commonly used tests to show the strength of an association are the risk ratio and the odds ratio. Both tell you how much more likely the outcome is to occur if the risk factor is present.

The risk ratio[61] is the probability of the outcome occurring in one group (e.g., treatment group) divided by the probability of the outcome occurring in the other group (e.g., placebo group).

Looking at our two-by-two table, the probability of an event in the group for which the risk factor is present is $a/(a + b)$ and the probability of an event in the group for which the risk factor is absent is $c/(c + d)$. Therefore, the risk ratio equals:

$$\text{risk ratio} = \frac{a/(a + b)}{c/(c + d)}$$

The risk ratio tells you how much more likely the outcome is to occur if the risk factor is present than if the risk factor is absent.

Let us compute the risk ratio of death due to diabetes from the data shown in Table 5.5.

$$\frac{47/726}{158/4206} = \frac{0.065}{0.038} = 1.71$$

This means that death is about 1.71 times more likely to occur among persons with diabetes than among persons without diabetes.

A risk ratio of <1.0 means that the outcome is less likely to occur if the risk factor is present. For example, if the risk ratio of death were 0.5 in persons who

---

[61] In some books the risk ratio will be referred to as the relative risk. It is best to think of the relative risk as a family of measures for comparing two groups. The risk ratio, the rate ratio, the prevalence ratio, and the hazard ratio are all forms of the relative risk. In general, it's best to use the more specific term.

Table 5.9. Association between diabetes and death

Diabetes	Death		Total
	Yes	No	
No	158 (77.1)	4048 (85.6)	4206 (85.3)
Yes	47 (22.9)	679 (14.4)	726 (14.7)
Total	205	4727	4932 (100)

Value are represented as n (%).

$\chi^2 = 11.48$; $P = 0.0007$.

Data from Bobrie, G., et al. Cardiovascular prognosis of "masked hypertension" detected by blood pressure self-management in elderly treated hypertensive patients. *J. Am. Med. Assoc.* 2004; 291: 1342–9.

exercise regularly then deaths would be expected to occur half as often among persons who exercise regularly compared to those who do not exercise regularly.

You may be wondering what would happen if you were to switch the order of the rows or columns. After all, our decision to set up the two-by-two table with the top row for the risk factor and the first column for the outcome having occurred is just convention.

In Table 5.9, I have switched the order of the rows from that of Table 5.5. Now the risk ratio is:

$$\frac{158/4206}{47/726} = \frac{0.038}{0.065} = 0.58$$

Which risk ratio (1.71 or 0.58) correctly expresses the association between diabetes and death? They both do. Saying that death is 1.71 times more likely among diabetics than persons without diabetes is mathematically equivalent to saying that death is 0.58 times less likely among persons without diabetes than diabetics. To prove that to yourself take the reciprocal of 1.71:

$$\frac{1}{1.71} = 0.58$$

> When the 95% confidence intervals of the risk ratio exclude 1, we say that there is a statistically significant increase (or decrease) in the risk of the outcome.

Risk ratios should always be reported with confidence intervals. By convention, if the 95% confidence intervals exclude 1, then we say that there is a statistically significant (at $P < 0.05$) increase (or decrease) in the risk of the outcome. When a higher degree of precision is needed you may report the 99% confidence intervals, and for exploratory studies you may want to report the 90% confidence intervals.

As the risk ratio is based on comparing the probabilities of an outcome (with and without the risk factor) it can also be used to calculate associations in cross-sectional studies. Although the formula for risk ratio is the same whether it is calculated for a prospective or cross-sectional study, when it is based on a cross-sectional study it should be referred to as the prevalence ratio. For example, Ebrahim and colleagues found that the prevalence of smoking was 11.8% among pregnant women and 23.6% among non-pregnant women. Therefore, the prevalence ratio is 0.5 (11.8%/23.6%).[62]

> Risk ratio cannot be used with case–control studies.

The risk ratio cannot, however, be used with case–control studies. The reason is that it is meaningless to speak of the probability of an outcome occurring in a case–control study. The probability of an outcome among the cases is 100% (that's what makes them cases) and the probability of an outcome among the controls is 0% (that's what makes them controls.) The probability of an outcome occurring in the entire sample (cases and controls) is determined by the investigator! If the investigator chooses one control per case then the probability of outcome in the sample will be 50%; if the investigator chooses three controls per case then the probability of outcome in the sample will be 25%, etc.

Instead, with case–control studies we use the odds ratio (OR). The odds ratio is the ratio of the odds of disease among those with the risk factor to the odds of disease among those without the risk factor.

Definition

The odds ratio is the ratio of the odds of disease among those with the risk factor to the odds of disease among those without the risk factor.

Looking back at Table 5.2, the odds of disease among those with the risk factor is a/b and the odds of disease among those without the risk factor is c/d. So the ratio is:

$$\frac{a/b}{c/d}$$

This can be rearranged to:

$$\frac{a}{b} \times \frac{d}{c} = \frac{a \times d}{b \times c}$$

As with risk ratios, the odds ratio should always be reported with confidence intervals.

A useful property of the odds ratio is that when an outcome is uncommon (<10–15%) the odds ratio approximates the risk ratio. For example, if we go back to the prospective study of diabetes as a risk factor for death (Table 5.5), the odds ratio would be:

$$\frac{47 \times 4048}{679 \times 158} = \frac{190,256}{107,282} = 1.77$$

Note that the odds ratio (1.77) is almost identical to the risk ratio (1.71)!

---

[62] Ebrahim, S.H., Floyd, R.L., Merritt, R.K., Decoufle, P., Holtzman, D. Trends in pregnancy-related smoking rates in the United States, 1987–1996. *J. Am. Med. Assoc.* 2000; 283: 361–6.

Table 5.10. Impact of cortical involvement on failure to improve among diabetic patients who received thrombolytic therapy

Cortical involvement	Failure to improve at 24 hours		Total
	Yes	No	
Yes	76 (50.5)	45 (49.5)	121
No	35 (16.0)	56 (84.0)	91
Total	111 (52)	101 (48)	212

Values are represented as *n* (%).
Odds ratio $(76 \times 56)/(45 \times 35) = 2.7$ (95% CI = 1.5–4.9).
Risk ratio $(76/121)/(35/91) = 1.6$ (95% CI = 1.2–2.2).
Data from Saposnik, G., et al. Lack of improvement in patients with acute stroke after treatment with thrombolytic therapy. *J. Am. Med. Assoc.* 2004; 292: 1839–44.

When the outcome is common in either group, the odds ratio no longer approximates the risk ratio. The difference between these two interpretations of the odds ratio can be seen in a prospective study of patients with stroke all of whom received thrombolytic therapy.[63] The investigators evaluated the impact of having cortical involvement on failure to improve at 24 hour.

Failure to improve was more common among those with cortical involvement (50.5%) than those without cortical involvement (16.0%) (Table 5.10). This is reflected in the risk ratio and odds ratio both being >1.0.

However, the sample was about evenly split between those who failed to improve (52%) and those who improved (48%). Since the outcome was common,[64] the odds ratio (2.7) is substantially higher than the risk ratio (1.6).

Investigators often report the odds ratio rather than the risk ratio when the frequency of the outcome is >10–15%. The reason is that many studies, including this one on the effect of cortical involvement on clinical improvement, perform multiple logistic regression, which produces odds ratios not risk ratios. In this study, the investigators performed multiple logistic regression so as to statistically adjust the odds ratios for age, sex, and stroke severity. The adjusted odds ratio was essentially the same as the unadjusted value (OR = 2.7; 95% CI = 1.4–5.2). Although the odds ratio does not approximate the risk ratio when the frequency is >10–15%, the odds ratio is still a valid measure of the association between a risk factor and an outcome.

Tip

To calculate the odds ratio when you have cells with no subjects in them, add 1/2 to each cell.

---

[63] Saposnik, G., Young, B., Silver, B., et al. Lack of improvement in patients with acute stroke after treatment with thrombolytic therapy. *J. Am. Med. Assoc.* 2004; 292: 1839–44.
[64] In determining whether the outcome occurs in <10–15% of the sample, use the less common state. In this study, the less common state is improvement (48%).

Table 5.11. Association between ethnicity and poor glycemic control

	Poor glycemic control ($HbA_{1c} > 10\%$)	
	Yes	No
African-American	2379 (28)	6117 (72)
Asian	1679 (22)	5953 (78)
Latino	1695 (27)	4584 (73)
Caucasians	7205 (18)	32,820 (82)

Values are represented as n (%).

$\chi^2 = 612; P < 0.0001$.

Data from Karter, A.J., et al. Ethnic disparities in diabetic complications in an insured population. *J. Am. Med. Assoc.* 2002; 287: 2519–27.

You may have noticed from the formula of the risk ratio and the odds ratio that they cannot be calculated if there is a cell with no subjects in it (because multiplying by zero will give you zero and dividing by zero is impossible). In such cases, you can add 1/2 to each of the cells so that you can calculate the odds ratio.

5.3 How do I test an association between a nominal variable and a dichotomous variable or between two nominal variables?

The categories of a nominal variable (e.g., ethnicity) have no numeric meaning (Section 2.10). To test the association between a nominal variable and a dichotomous variable or to test the association between two nominal variables use a chi-squared statistic. As chi-squared compares the expected number of subjects to the observed number of subjects in each cell, the test is unaffected by the order of the categories.

Contingency tables for assessing an association involving a nominal variable are generally called *r*-by-*c* (row by column) tables. More specifically, Table 5.11, which assesses the association between ethnicity and poor glycemic control ($HbA_{1c} > 10\%$) among persons with diabetes,[65] is a four-by-two table, because it has four rows and two columns.

The significant chi-squared tells you that the differences in glycemic control across ethnicities are unlikely to have occurred by chance. The chi-squared does *not* tell you which groups are significantly different from one another – only that the overall pattern is significantly different from what would have been expected by chance.

Looking at the percentages in Table 5.11 you can tell that poor glycemic control is most common among African-American patients. But you cannot say

---

[65] Karter, A.J., Ferrara, A., Liu, J.Y., Moffet, H.H., Ackerson, L.M., Selby, J.V. Ethnic disparities in diabetic complications in an insured population. *J. Am. Med. Assoc.* 2002; 287: 2519–27.

Table 5.12. Association between African-American ethnicity and poor glycemic control

	Poor glycemic control ($HbA_{1c} > 10\%$)	
	Yes	No
African-American	2379 (28)	6117 (72)
All other ethnicities	10,579 (20)	43,357 (80)

Values are represented as n (%).
$\chi^2 = 314; P < 0.0001$.

Table 5.13. Comparison of glycemic control among African-Americans and Latinos

	Poor glycemic control ($HbA_{1c} > 10\%$)	
	Yes	No
African-American	2379 (28)	6117 (72)
Latino	1695 (27)	4584 (73)

Values are represented as n (%).
$\chi^2 = 1.8; P = 0.18$.

from Table 5.11 whether poor glycemic control is significantly more common among African-Americans than among persons of other ethnicities.

To determine if poor glycemic control is significantly more common among African-Americans you would need to collapse Table 5.11 into a two-by-two table comparing African-Americans to persons of all other ethnicities (Table 5.12).

As indicated by the large chi-squared and the small P-value, poor glycemic control is more common among African-Americans than among non-African-Americans. But is poor glycemic control significantly more common among African-Americans than Latinos? You cannot answer this from either Tables 5.11 or 5.12. To answer this you would need to directly compare these two groups as shown in Table 5.13.

As you can see the chi-squared value is small and the P-value is >0.05. The difference in glycemic control between African-Americans and Latinos is not statistically significant.

In making pairwise comparisons such as those shown in Table 5.13, it is important to avoid capitalizing on chance. Specifically, it stands to reason that if you have four groups and you compare the highest group to the lowest group you are more likely to find a statistical difference than if you compare the four groups to each other. For this reason, if the overall chi-squared is not significant, pairwise

Tip

Be wary of pairwise comparisons if the overall chi-squared is not statistically significant.

comparisons should be interpreted very cautiously: they may not represent a true difference. If you are making multiple pairwise comparisons you should also set a more stringent P-value to avoid capitalizing on chance (Section 5.6.A).

As with two-by-two table (Section 5.2), if any of the cells of an r-by-c table are expected to have fewer than 5 subjects you need to use an exact test. There is an extension of the Fisher's exact test for r-by-c tables. As it is computationally difficult not all statistical packages produce exact tests for contingency tables bigger than two-by-two. However, special statistical programs for computing exact tests for r-by-c tables are available.[66]

Alternatively, when faced with an expected cell frequency of <5 subjects you can collapse the rows or columns. For example, in the case of ethnicity you may have to resort to three categories instead of four (e.g., Caucasian, African-Americans, others). Or if you will still have an expected cell frequency of <5, collapse the categories even further (e.g., Caucasian versus non-Caucasians). Alternatively, you could drop subjects of uncommon ethnicities from the analysis. Of course, whenever you collapse categories or drop subjects, information is lost. Ultimately, the best solution is to sample from a more diverse population!

5.4 How do I test an association involving an interval variable? (When do I use parametric statistics versus non-parametric statistics?)

With interval variables, the type of bivariate analysis you should perform depends on whether the variable fulfills the assumptions of normality and equal variance.

In Section 4.2, I suggested several univariate methods of assessing whether a variable has a normal distribution. When you are performing bivariate analyses, the dependent variable (outcome) must have a normal distribution at *each* value of your independent variable (risk factor) (rather than at all values of the independent variable taken together). Also, the spread of values from the mean of the outcome should be equal at each value of your independent variable (assumption of equal variance).

For example, Figure 5.1(a) shows a hypothetical distribution of resting pulse rate for three groups: marathon runners, moderate exercisers, and couch potatoes. Note that the pulse for each of three groups forms a bell-shaped curve, indicating that the variable has a normal distribution at each value of the independent variable. Also note that even though all three distributions are bell-shaped, the values are very different: the marathon runners have substantially slower pulses than the couch potatoes (the dotted line equals the mean of each group). Finally, note that

> **Definition**
>
> Equal variance means that the spread of values from the mean of the outcome is equal for each value of the independent variable.

---

[66] If your software does not produce exact tests for r-by-c tables (or you need an exact test for a different reason, such as exact confidence intervals for an odds ratio) see: www.statsdirect.com. They offer a free trial of the product.

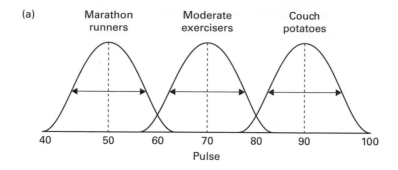

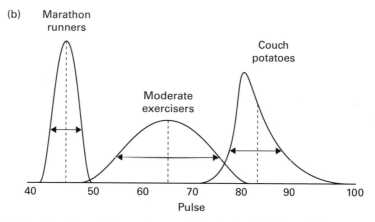

Figure 5.1   Plots of an interval dependent variable (pulse) for three different groups. (a) The assumptions of normal distribution and equal variance are fulfilled because for all three groups (marathon runners, moderate exercisers, and couch potatoes) the curves are bell-shaped and the spread from the mean (indicated by arrows) is equal. (b) These assumptions are not met. The assumption of normal distribution is violated because the distribution of values for couch potatoes is not bell-shaped. The equal variance assumption is invalid because the spread of values from the mean is different for the different groups.

the distribution of pulse rates for all three groups fulfills the assumptions of equal variance – the spread of values from the mean (indicated by arrows) is equal for the different groups.

In Figure 5.1(b), the hypothetical distributions of pulse rate for the three groups do not fulfill the assumptions of normality and equal variance. Although the distribution of values for the runners and the moderate exercisers are normal, the distribution for couch potatoes is skewed to the right. Also the equal variance assumption is invalid because the spread of values from the mean is different for the different groups.

If you are testing the association of an interval risk factor with an interval outcome, it may be unwieldy to check whether the assumptions of normality

Tip

When assessing the association between an interval risk factor and an interval outcome check the assumptions of normality and equal variance by grouping the risk factor into a few categories.

Tip

If your sample size is >100, you can treat your interval variables as if they were normally distributed in your analyses.

and equal variance are met if there are a lot of possible values for the risk factor. In such cases, recode the risk factor into a few groups so that you can test the assumption. For example, if you are testing the association of weight with age, you could group age into four categories: 20–39 years, 40–59 years, 60–79 years, 80 or greater years of age.[67]

As you can see, testing each of your interval independent variables to see if it fulfills the assumptions of normality and equal variance with your outcome variable would be very tedious. I am happy to report that if your sample size is large (>100), and there are no unduly influential points (an observation that has a disproportionate impact on the bivariate or multivariable analysis) than you can treat your interval variables as if they were normally distributed in your analyses.[68] If your sample size is <100 and your interval variable does not fulfill the assumptions of normality, then use non-parametric statistics to analyse it.

A large sample size does not exempt your data from having to fulfill the assumptions of equal variance. Formal tests for equal variance are available (Section 5.5.A), however, because these tests can give false reassurance when the sample size is small, some authors recommend against using them.[69] When performing t-tests, unequal variances can be dealt with by calculating a t-test with unequal variances (Section 5.5.A). In the case of analysis of variance (ANOVA), unequal variances will generally result in decreasing the power of your analysis to demonstrate an association between the variables.

Non-parametric statistics are based on the rankings of each subject within the sample. Subjects are ranked in ascending or descending order based on their values on a particular variable.

For example, Vitovski and colleagues measured IgA1 protease activity by strains of *Haemophilus influenzae*.[70] IgA1 proteases impede the body's ability to defend itself against bacteria and therefore differences in IgA1 protease activity may explain some of the differences in the virulence of *Haemophilus influenzae*.

The IgA1 activity levels of *Haemophilus influenzae* was not normal, but was right-skewed. Due to this the investigators used rank statistics to analyse the data. To illustrate how to calculate ranks I have ordered the values of the 19 strains of *Haemophilus influenzae* from throat swabs of asymptomatic carriers

---

[67] Although it is always good to begin testing for normality and equal variance by drawing histograms of your interval data, there are a number of more sophisticated methods for testing these assumptions. For an excellent review of using residuals to verify these assumptions see: Glantz, S.A., Slinker, B.K. *Primer of Applied Regression and Analysis of Variance*. New York: McGraw-Hill, pp. 125–77. For tests of homogeneity of variances when performing t-tests or ANOVA, see Section 5.5.A.

[68] We can do this because of the central limit theorem; see: Rosner, B. *Fundamentals of Biostatistics* (5th edition). Pacific Grove: Duxbury, 2000, pp. 174–6.

[69] Vittinghoff, E., Glidden, D.V., Shiboski, S.C., McCulloch, C.E. *Regression Methods in Biostatistics*. New York: Springer, 2005, pp. 33–5, 119.

[70] Vitovski, S., Dunkin, K.T., Howard, A.J., Sayers, J.R. Nontypeable *Haemophilus influenzae* in carriage and disease: a difference in IgA1 protease activity levels. *J. Am. Med. Assoc.* 2002; 287: 1699–705.

Table 5.14. IgA1 protease activity 19 different strains of *Haemophilus influenzae* isolated from throat swabs of asymptomatic carriers

Strain	IgA1 protease activity	Rank
C9	ND*	2.5
C11	ND	2.5
94C.52	ND	2.5
94C.255	ND	2.5
C12	10	5
C3	20	7
C4	20	7
94C.225	20	7
C7	30	9.5
94C.238	30	9.5
C1	40	11.5
94C.288	40	11.5
C5	50	13
94C.295	60	14
C10	120	15.5
94C.47	120	15.5
C8	130	17
C2	160	18
94C.230	210	19

*ND = non-detectable.

Data from Vitovski, S., et al. Nontypeable *Haemophilus influenzae* in carriage and disease: a difference in IgA1 protease activity levels. *J. Am. Med. Assoc.* 2002; 287: 1699–705.

from lowest to highest activity (column 2, Table 5.14) and the ranks of the 19 strains (column 3, Table 5.14). When there are ties, as there are in Table 5.14, each tied observation receives the average of the ranks on which they tie. For example, there are four strains for which IgA1 protease activity was not detectable. The average of these four tied rankings is 2.5 [(1 + 2 + 3 + 4)/4)].

One of the advantages to ranking is that we do not have to assign a numeric value of zero to those observations that are undetectable (these may strains produce some IgA1 protease activity but the assay is not sensitive enough to detect it). We know, however, that the ranking would be less than the strains that produced activity at the level of 10.

With non-parametric statistics only the rankings (column 3) are used in calculating the test. The actual values (column 2) play no role in determining the statistics or the *P*-value. Besides being useful for interval variables that violate

> Non-parametric statistics are based on the rankings of each subject and do not require a normal distribution.

Table 5.15. Comparison of parametric and non-parametric statistics for testing bivariate associations

Type of variables	If interval variable is:	
	Parametric	Non-parametric
Dichotomous variable and an interval variable	*t*-test	Mann-Whitney test
Nominal variable and an interval variable	ANOVA	Kruskal–Wallis test
Correction for multiple pairwise comparisons of interval variables	Bonferroni	Dunn's test
Two interval variables	Pearson's correlation coefficient, linear regression	Spearman's rank correlation coefficient

the assumptions of normality and/or equal variance, non-parametric statistics are also very useful for analyzing ordinal variables. Since non-parametric statistics are based on ranks, it does not matter that there is not an equal difference between the levels of the scale.

You might ask why not just use non-parametric statistics to analyse all associations involving an interval variable. Then you would not need to check the assumptions of normality and equal variance, and you could analyse your interval and ordinal variables in the same way. The answer is that non-parametric statistics are not as powerful as parametric statistics. A ballpark estimate is that you lose about 10% of power if you analyse a parametric variable using non-parametric statistics.

> Non-parametric statistics are not as powerful as parametric statistics.

Table 5.15 compares the parametric and non-parametric statistics for testing bivariate associations. Greater detail is provided in Sections 5.5 and 5.6.

In some cases, you may be able to transform a non-normally distributed interval variable so that it will have a normal distribution. When this is possible, it's an excellent strategy because it enables you to use the more powerful parametric statistics. For example, a variable with a skewed distribution to the right (Figure 4.2) will often approximate a bell-shaped curve if you transform it by taking the logarithm of each subject's value:

new variable = logarithm (non-normally distributed interval variable)

One problem with this approach is that it may make your results less accessible to clinical readers. Physicians, for example, are not used to thinking in terms of the impact of the logarithm of a patient's blood pressure on risk of stroke. But the bigger problem is that for many variables there is no mathematical transformation that normalizes the distribution.

> Variables can be dichotomized using a natural cut-off, median split, or comparison of extreme categories.

You can also incorporate a non-normally distributed interval variable into a parametric analysis by dichotomizing it. This is usually done in one of three ways: at a natural cut-off, a median split, or a comparison of extreme categories.

If the variable has a cut-off point that is clinically useful, such as diastolic blood pressure of <90 mmHg versus 90 mmHg or more, using this cut-off for your study will make sense to clinical readers. When there is no natural cut-off, median splits (Section 3.6.A) are a good choice because they will provide you a near equal division of your sample (unless you have a large number of subjects exactly at the median). This will maximize the statistical power of your analysis. Finally, in some circumstances authors are interested in examining subjects with extreme values on an interval variable. For example, investigators may be interested in comparing the diets of persons with the highest and lowest choles-terol levels. This strategy may highlight differences between groups that might otherwise be diluted by including many people who are just above or just below the median. A downside of this strategy is that it diminishes sample size because the people in the middle (those with average values on the variable) are not included in the analysis.

One method not to use in dividing your sample is to choose the cut-off based on what cut-off would result in the finding you are looking for! Choosing a cut-off based on the data capitalizes on chance and makes your P-values meaning-less. Also remember that when you dichotomize an interval variable, you lose a lot of valuable information. In terms of risk of stroke, having a diastolic blood pressure of 110 mmHg is very different than having a diastolic blood pressure of 91 mmHg even though both could be coded as >90 mmHg.

> **Tip**
>
> Avoid dichotomizing interval variables because you will lose valuable information.

5.5　How do I test an association of a dichotomous variable with an interval variable?

5.5.A　Association of a dichotomous variable with a normally distributed interval variable

When determining the association between a dichotomous variable and a nor-mally distributed interval variable use the (Student's) t-test.

The t-test is essentially a comparison of the means of the two groups. We seek to disprove the null hypothesis; that is, that there is no difference between the two means.

The t-test is calculated as the difference between the two means divided by the standard error of that difference:

> **Tip**
>
> Use the t-test to compare the means of two groups.

$$t = \frac{\text{mean of sample 1} - \text{mean of sample 2}}{\text{standard error of difference between mean 1 and mean 2}}$$

With a sample size of at least 60 subjects a t-value of 2.0 will be statistically significant at the <0.05 threshold. A t-value of 2.0 or greater is an intuitively meaningful threshold. It signifies that the difference between the means of the two groups is at least twice the size of the error of the measurement of that difference.

If the difference between the means is small or if the error in the measurement of the difference is large compared to the difference in the means, then the *t*-value will not reach statistical significance.

From the formula you can also see why the *t*-test may not be valid for variables with non-normal distributions. If the mean is not an accurate measurement of the center of the distribution, then a test based on the comparison of means may not be valid.

The actual *P*-value associated with a given *t*-value will depend on the degrees of freedom. For a *t*-test, the degrees of freedom are:

$$\text{degrees of freedom} = \text{sample size group A} + \text{sample size group B} - 2$$

The *t*-test formula above is only accurate when the variances of the two groups are equal (Section 5.4). Unequal variance is especially a problem when the sample sizes are unequal and the smaller sample is associated with the larger variance.

When the variances are unequal, you will need to perform a *t*-test for unequal variances. How do you determine whether or not the variances are equal?

> When comparing the means of two groups check to see if the variances are equal by using Levene's test.

There are several tests available for calculating whether the variances are equal. A commonly used test of the equality of variances is Bartlett's test. However, it is inaccurate when the distribution of the data are non-normal. Levene's test is less sensitive to deviations from normality and only a little less powerful than Bartlett's test. It tests the null hypothesis that the variances are equal. If the *P*-value for the *F* is <0.05 then you should reject the null hypothesis and assume that the variances are unequal.[71]

Fortunately, most statistical software packages automatically calculate the *t*-value two ways: assuming equal and unequal variances. If the variances are equal report the value of the *t*-test assuming equal variance. If the variances are unequal report the value of the *t*-test assuming unequal variance.

A limitation of the *t*-test is that it does not give the reader direct information on the numeric difference between the two groups. A useful method of quantifying the difference between two groups is to calculate the numeric difference between the two means (i.e., mean difference = mean 1 − mean 2) and the 95% confidence interval of that difference.[72] If the 95% confidence interval excludes zero then the difference between the means would be considered statistically significant.

---

[71] For more on these two tests of homogeneity of variance see: Glantz, S.A., Slinker, B.K. *Primer of Applied Regression and Analysis of Variance.* New York: McGraw-Hill, pp. 308–9.

[72] For the formulas to calculate the confidence intervals of the difference of the mean see: Glantz, S.A. *Primer of Biostatistics* (5th edition). New York: McGraw-Hill, 2002, pp. 200–9.

Table 5.16. Differences in weight loss (at 6 months) with two different diets

Low carbohydrate diet, kg	Low fat diet, kg	Mean difference (95% CI), kg
5.8	1.9	3.9 (1.6–6.3)

Data from Samaha, F.F., et al. A low-carbohydrate as compared with a low-fat diet in severe obesity. *New Engl. J. Med.* 2003; 348: 2074–81.

This works, especially well with variables measured in clinically meaningful metrics such as weight.

For example, Samaha and colleagues compared weight loss among obese subjects randomized to one of two different diets (Table 5.16).[73] The difference in weight loss between the two diets (3.9 kg) and the 95% confidence interval of that difference (1.6–6.3 kg) give you a much better understanding of the difference between these two diets than a "*t*"- or "*P*"-value ever could.

> **Tip**
>
> Report the mean difference with its confidence interval, not just the "*t*"- or "*P*"-value.

5.5.B Association of a dichotomous variable with a non-normally distributed interval variable

When determining the association of a dichotomous variable with a non-normally distributed interval variable, use the Mann-Whitney test (also known as the Mann-Whitney *U*-test, the Mann-Whitney rank sum test, and the Wilcoxon rank sum test[74]). The Mann-Whitney test is a comparison of the rankings of two groups.

In Section 5.4, I showed how to rank a group of observations (Table 5.14). To compare two groups we rank the observations from the lowest to the highest value without regard to which group they are in. To illustrate, let us continue with the example of IgA1 protease activity by strains of *Haemophilus influenzae*.

In Table 5.17, I have ordered the observations of IgA1 protease activity of two groups: strains collected from asymptomatic carriers (same as Table 5.14) and strains from the sputum of symptomatic patients. Having ordered them from highest to lowest, I can then easily rank them.

Note that the rankings of the strains from asymptomatic carriers are different in Table 5.17 than in Table 5.14. That's because in Table 5.14, I was ranking the observations of only one group, while for Table 5.17, I am ranking the observations of two groups.[75]

> **Tip**
>
> Use the Mann-Whitney test to compare two groups on a non-normally distributed interval variable.

---

[73] Samaha, F.F., Iqbal, N., Seshadri, P. et al. A low-carbohydrate as compared with a low-fat diet in severe obesity. *New Engl. J. Med.* 2003; 348: 2074–81.

[74] The Wilcoxon test (Section 5.9) and the Wilcoxon signed rank test (Section 5.10) are different from each other and different than the Wilcoxon rank sum test.

[75] If you wish to calculate a Mann-Whitney test, and have not already entered your data into a statistical package that performs this test, go to: http://eatworms.swmed.edu/~leon/stats/utest.html

Table 5.17. IgA1 protease activity of *Haemophilus influenzae* strains from asymptomatic carriers and symptomatic persons

	Asymptomatic carriers (throat swabs)			Symptomatic persons (sputum samples)	
Strain	IgA1 protease activity	Rank	Strain	IgA1 activity	Rank
C9	ND*	3.5	8,625	ND	3.5
C11	ND	3.5	77,688	ND	3.5
94C.52	ND	3.5	77,321	40	14.5
94C.255	ND	3.5	77,332	40	14.5
C12	10	7	77,417	50	17.5
C3	20	9	2,005	70	20
C4	20	9	7,244	90	21
94C.225	20	9	6,350	100	22
C7	30	11.5	1,428	120	24
94C.238	30	11.5	7,693	130	26.5
C1	40	14.5	77,459	190	29.5
94C.288	40	14.5	5,220	190	29.5
C5	50	17.5	77,423	220	32
94C.295	60	19	77,462	240	33
C10	120	24	77,421	300	34
94C.47	120	24	1,958	320	35
C8	130	26.5	77,454	380	36
C2	160	28	6,338	430	37
94C.230	210	31	8,304	570	38
			77,412	600	39
Sum of ranks		270			510

*ND = non-detectable.

Data from Vitovski, S., et al. Nontypeable *Haemophilus influenzae* in carriage and disease: a difference in IgA1 protease activity levels. *J. Am. Med. Assoc.* 2002; 287: 1699–705.

Having ranked the observations, I next sum the ranks of the two samples. Given that the two groups have approximately the same number of observations, we would expect that the sum of the rankings would be about equal in the two groups assuming that there were no association between IgA1 protease activity and whether the strain was cultured from an asymptomatic carrier or a symptomatic person. As you can see, the sum of the rankings of the asymptomatic carriers is, in fact, much smaller.

For any two samples, we can determine the probability of obtaining a particular sum of the rankings for the smaller group under the assumption that there is no difference between the two groups. If the generated sum of the rankings of the smaller group is much higher (or lower) then the sum you would expect if there is no difference between the two groups, then you can reject the null hypothesis and conclude that there is a difference between the two groups. This is the case with Table 5.17. The P-value associated with the Mann-Whitney test is $P < 0.01$.

With small sample sizes the Mann-Whitney test is much weaker than the t-test. In fact, if you have seven or few data points (both groups combined), the Mann-Whitney test will not be statistically significant at the threshold of $P = 0.05$ (two-tailed test) no matter how great the differences are between the two groups.[76]

5.6 How do I test an association of a nominal variable with an interval variable?

5.6.A Association of a nominal variable with a normally distributed interval variable (comparison of three or more means)

> **Tip**
>
> Use ANOVA to compare three or more means.

Testing the association of a nominal variable with an interval parametric variable (e.g., the association of ethnicity and blood pressure) is similar to testing the association of a dichotomous variable with an interval parametric variable (e.g., the association of sex and blood pressure). In both situations you are comparing means. The difference is that with a nominal variable, there are three or more groups. In such situations, use ANOVA.

An ANOVA tests the null hypothesis that there is no difference in the means of the different groups; in other words, any differences between the means are due to random variation.

The "variance" in the name refers to the difference between the values of the individual subjects and the mean.[77] There are two means to consider: the mean of the whole sample and the mean of each group. The "between-groups" variance is based on the differences between the subjects and the overall mean. The "within-group" variance is based on the differences between the group members and the group mean.

ANOVA produces an F-value. The F-value is the ratio of the between-groups variance to the within-groups variance.

$$F = \frac{\text{between-groups variance (variance calculated based on the entire sample)}}{\text{within-groups variance (variance calculated separately for each group)}}$$

---

[76] Motulsky H. *Intuitive Biostatistics.* Oxford: Oxford University Press, 1995, pp. 221–4.
[77] For an excellent (and free) explanation of ANOVA, see Statsoft an electronic textbook at: (http://www.statsoft.com/textbook/stanman.html.)

If the means of the groups are very different then the variance calculated based on the mean of the entire sample (between-groups variance) will be larger than the variance when it is calculated separately for each group (within-groups variance). This will result in a large F-value and (assuming a large enough sample) a small P-value. With a small P-value you can reject the null hypothesis that the group means are the same.

To compute a P-value for the F-value you need to determine the degrees of freedom for the numerator (the between-groups variance) and for the denominator (within-groups variance). For the numerator, the degrees of freedom is the number of groups minus 1. For the denominator, the degrees of freedom is the total sample size minus the number of groups.

In addition to assuming that the interval variable is normally distributed for each of the groups, ANOVA assumes that the observations of the groups have equal variance (Section 5.4). You can check for equal variance using the Levene test.[78] If there are significant departures from equal variance you can use the Kruskal–Wallis test, a test based on ranks, to compare the groups (Section 5.6.B). With ranks, unequal variance of the original scores is not an issue.

One important limitation of ANOVA is that it does not indicate where the difference lies. A large F just tells you that you can reject the null hypothesis that *all* the means are the same. In the case of a comparison of three groups A, B, and C, there are a total of seven possible ways that the groups may differ from one another:

A is different than B (but not different than C)
A is different than C (but not different than B)
B is different than C (but not different than A)
A is different from both B and C (which are not different from one another)
B is different from both A and C (which are not different from one another)
C is different from both A and B (which are not different from one another)
A and B and C are all different from one another

To detect where the actual differences lie, you will need to perform pairwise comparisons of the groups using a t-test. You are already familiar with the t-test from the previous section. The important difference is that when you use the t-test for pairwise comparisons you are performing multiple comparisons.

When making multiple comparisons you should set a more stringent criteria (i.e., a lower P-value) before rejecting the null hypothesis. The reason is that if we set our threshold for rejecting the null hypothesis at $P = 0.05$, we are accepting that there is a 5% chance that the null hypothesis is correct even though we have

---

[78] The Levene test is explained in Section 5.5.A. However, as explained in reference 18 limitations of these tests lead some authors to recommend against using them.

rejected it (see type I error, Section 2.7). If we perform three possible pairwise comparisons (A versus B; B versus C; A versus C) and reject the null hypothesis all three times at the threshold of $P = 0.05$, then we are accepting a 0.15 probability (0.05×3) that we are incorrectly rejecting the null hypothesis at least once.

To avoid this problem set a more stringent P-value when making multiple comparisons. The most commonly used method for adjusting the significance level for multiple pairwise comparisons is the Bonferroni correction. It is very straightforward. You simply divide the probability threshold that you would use if you were performing a single test (usually 0.05) by the number of pairwise comparisons you are performing.

> **Tip**
>
> When making multiple pairwise comparisons, set a more stringent P-value to avoid capitalizing on chance.

Bonferroni correction:

$$\frac{\text{significance level assuming you are performing a single test}}{\text{number of pairwise comparisons you are performing}} = \text{new more stringent } P\text{-value}$$

For example, if you are performing three pairwise comparisons, you would reject the null hypothesis only if $P \leq 0.017$ ($0.05/3 = 0.017$). If you were performing four pairwise comparisons, you would reject the null hypothesis only if $P \leq 0.013$ ($0.05/4 = 0.013$).

The Bonferroni correction has a number of advantages. It is easy to compute and very flexible. Since it is a correction of the P-value (rather than of the statistic) you can use it anytime you are making multiple comparisons. It can be used with multiple comparisons based on t-tests, or chi-squared analyses, or Kaplan–Meier curves. It can be used with paired or unpaired data, etc.

On the other hand, it is a conservative adjustment, especially as the number of comparisons increase. In such cases you may wish to consider one of the more sophisticated approaches to adjusting for multiple pairwise comparisons.[79]

5.6.B Association of a nominal variable with a non-normally distributed interval variable (comparison of the rankings of three or more groups)

To assess the association of a nominal variable with a non-normally distributed interval variable use the Kruskal–Wallis test. The Kruskal–Wallis test is a comparison of the rankings of three or more groups.

---

[79] Glantz, S.A. *Primer of Biostatistics* (5th edition). New York: McGraw-Hill, 2002, pp. 89–107; Motulsky H. *Intuitive Biostatistics.* Oxford: Oxford University Press, 1995, pp. 259.

Table 5.18. Association of myeloperoxidase index with angina

Myeloperoxidase index*	Unstable angina, left coronary lesion ($n = 24$)	Unstable angina, right coronary lesion ($n = 9$)	Chronic stable angina ($n = 13$)	Variant angina ($n = 13$)	Controls ($n = 6$)
Median	−6.4	−6.6	0.6	−0.4	−0.2
Range	−15.8 – −0.4	−13.9 – −4.0	−4.0 – 8.9	−9.4 – 11.0	−4.6 – 4.6

* Sampled from great cardiac vein.

Data from Buffon, A., et al. Widespread coronary inflammation in unstable angina. *New Engl. J. Med.* 2002; 347: 5–12.

> **Tip**
>
> Use the Kruskal–Wallis test to compare three or more groups on a non-normally distributed interval variable.

Similar to the Mann-Whitney test, the Kruskal–Wallis test is based on ranking subjects from lowest to highest on the value of interest and then summing the ranks of each group. If there is no difference between the groups and the sample size is the same then the sum of the ranks for the groups should be about the same. If there is a large difference, the Kruskal–Wallis H-value (which approximates a chi-squared distribution) will be large and the P-value will be small. You can then reject the null hypothesis and consider the alternative hypothesis that the groups are different.

As with the F-test of ANOVA, knowing that the groups differ based on the Kruskal–Wallis test does not tell you where the differences lie. To do this most investigators use Dunn's test, because other available tests (variants of the Student–Newman–Keuls and Dunnett's test) require that the groups have an equal sample size, a condition rarely met in clinical studies.[80] In calculating the P-value, Dunn's test takes into account the number of comparisons you are making.

> **Tip**
>
> Use Dunn's test to perform pairwise comparisons of non-normally distributed interval variables.

For example, Buffon and colleagues studied the relationship between coronary inflammation and unstable angina.[81] The investigators measured the neutrophil myeloperoxidase index in the cardiac circulations. Low levels of the index are associated with activation of neutrophils, indicating inflammation. The index is not normally distributed. There were five different groups with unequal sample sizes (Table 5.18).

Since the data are not normally distributed, the investigators show the median and the range rather than the mean and standard deviation. As you can see from looking at the medians, the index was strongly negative for patients with unstable angina (whether they had a left or a right coronary lesion) but was close to zero for patients with chronic stable angina, variant angina, and for control patients.

---

[80] Glantz, S.A. *Primer of Biostatistics* (5th edition). New York: McGraw-Hill, 2002, p. 366.

[81] Buffon, A., Biasucci, L.M., Liuzzo, G., et al. Widespread coronary inflammation in unstable angina. *New Engl. J. Med.* 2002; 347: 5–12.

Table 5.19. Pairwise comparisons of myeloperoxidase index levels

Comparison	Versus	P-value
Unstable angina with left coronary lesion	Chronic stable angina	<0.001
Unstable angina with left coronary lesion	Variant angina	0.004
Unstable angina with left coronary lesion	Controls	0.004
Unstable angina with a right coronary lesion	Chronic stable angina	<0.001
Unstable angina with a right coronary lesion	Variant angina	0.002
Unstable angina with a right coronary lesion	Controls	0.001

Data from Buffon, A., et al. Widespread coronary inflammation in unstable angina. *New Engl. J. Med.* 2002; 347: 5–12.

The results of pairwise comparisons using Dunn's test are shown in Table 5.19. Note that the authors did not compare the two groups with unstable angina to each other or the three groups without unstable angina to each other because the hypothesis of the study is that unstable angina leads to activation of neutrophils and low levels of the index. No clinically meaningful differences were expected within the group of patients with unstable angina or within the group of patients without stable angina.

5.7 How do I test an association between two interval variables? (How do I determine if an association is linear?)

> **Tip**
>
> Always plot interval variables using a scatterplot before performing statistical analysis.

The first step in evaluating an association between two interval variables is to perform a scatterplot. A scatterplot will allow you to determine the nature of the relationship between the two variables.

For example, Uren and colleagues studied the relationship between the severity of coronary artery stenosis and myocardial blood flow.[82] They measured the coronary vasodilator reserve (the ratio of myocardial blood flow during hyperemia to flow at baseline) for 35 patients with single-vessel coronary artery disease. If a vessel is unable to dilate the patient will experience ischemia (insufficient blood to the heart) with exertion.

Figure 5.2 shows how the minimal luminal diameter (*x*-axis) is related to the coronary vasodilator reserve (*y*-axis). Each circle represents a subject. When the diameter of the lumen is <1, the vessel has no ability to dilate (a coronary

---

[82] Uren, N.G., Melin, J.A., De Bruyne, B., Wijns, W., Baudhuin, T., Camici, P.G. Relation between myocardial blood flow and the severity of coronary-artery stenosis. *New Engl. J. Med.* 1994; 330: 1782–8.

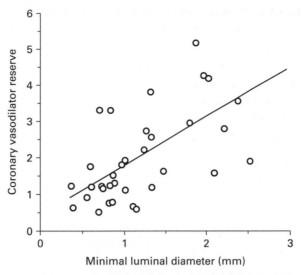

Figure 5.2

Strong linear association between minimal luminal diameter and coronary vasodilator reserve. Reprinted with permission from Uren, N.G., et al. Relation between myocardial blood flow and the severity of coronary artery stenosis. *New Engl. J. Med.* 1994; 330: 1782–8. Copyright 1994 Massachusetts Medical Society.

vasodilator reserve of 1 indicates no increase in flow with hyperemia). As the luminal diameter increases, the reserve also increases in a linear fashion.

When there is a linear association, Pearson's correlation coefficient and linear regression (Section 5.7.A) can be used to quantify that relationship for parametric variables; Spearman's rank correlation can be used for non-normally distributed interval variables (Section 5.7.B).

However, interval variables may be associated with one another in non-linear ways. For example, Glynn and colleagues found a **U**-shaped relationship between diastolic blood pressure and cognitive function (Figure 5.3).[83] Specifically, extremely low and extremely high blood pressures were associated with worsened cognitive function (measured by the square root of the number of errors made on a mental status questionnaire).

If you are having trouble seeing the **U**-shaped relationship from the dots, cover the graph with a piece of paper and then slide it across the plot from right to left (from a diastolic blood pressure of 40 mmHg to a diastolic blood pressure of

---

[83] Glynn, R.J., Beckett, L.A., Hebert, L.E., Morris, M.C., Scherr, P.A., Evans, D.A. Current and remote blood pressure and cognitive decline. *J. Am. Med. Assoc.* 1999; 281: 438–45.

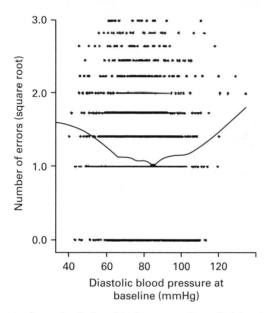

Figure 5.3

U-shaped relationship between diastolic blood pressure and cognitive function (measured by the square root of the number of errors made). Reprinted with permission from Glynn, R.J., et al. Current and remote blood pressure and cognitive decline. *J. Am. Med. Assoc.* 1999; 281: 438–45. Copyright 1999 American Medical Association. All rights reserved.

120 mmHg). Note that a much higher proportion of the dots are above 1.0 among persons with low blood pressure than among the subjects with intermediate blood pressures (in the middle of the plot). When you get to the far right of the plot (where the values are for the subjects with high blood pressures), you again see a much higher proportion of the dots above 1.0 than in the middle of the plot.

U-shaped relationships may also be upside down such that higher values are seen in the middle. A **J**-shaped association is essentially the same as a **U**-shaped association, except you are missing part of one of the legs of the **U**. A **J**-shaped association may also be reversed so the shorter leg is to the right of the longer leg.

A threshold relationship exists when changes in the independent variable at certain points in the scale result in changes in the outcome while changes at other points in the scale changes do not (or only modestly) affect the outcome. For example, as shown in Figure 5.4 there is a threshold association between lifetime blood lead level and IQ (as measured by the Stanford–Binet Intelligence Test score).[84] As blood lead levels increase, IQ decreases in a linear fashion until

---

[84] Canfield, R.L., Hendeerson, C.R., Cory-Slechta, D.A., Cox, C., Jusko, T.A., Lanphear, B.P. Intellectual impairment in children with blood lead concentrations below 10 μg per deciliter. *New Engl. J. Med.* 2003; 348: 1517–26.

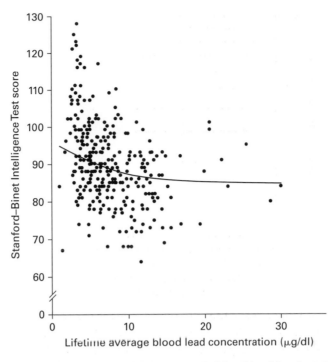

Figure 5.4   IQ decreases linearly with increases in blood lead level up to 10 μg/dl; after this threshold, IQ decreases only slightly with increases in blood lead level. Reprinted with permission from Canfield, R.L., et al. Intellectual impairment in children with blood lead concentrations below 10 μg per deciliter. *New Engl. J. Med.* 2003; 348: 1517–26. Copyright 2003 Massachusetts Medical Society. All rights reserved.

the lead level reaches about 10 μg/dl. After this point, higher lead levels result in only modest decreases in IQ. These results are of great public health significance. Prior to this study, most childhood lead programs focused on identifying children with high blood lead concentrations (10 μg/dl or above), thereby missing a large number of children who may be harmed by moderate lead levels.

There are countless non-linear relationships possible between two interval variables. If you detect a non-linear relationship association between two variables you will need to either transform one or both of the variables so that the association between them becomes linear or use more sophisticated methods for analyzing non-linear associations such as spline functions.[85]

---

[85] See: Harrell, F.E. *Regression Modeling Strategies: With Applications to Linear Models, Logistic Regression, and Survival Analysis.* New York: Springer-Verlag, 2001, pp. 18–24; Katz, M.H. *Multivariable Analysis: A Practical Guide for Clinicians* (2nd edition). Cambridge University Press, 2005, 46–51.

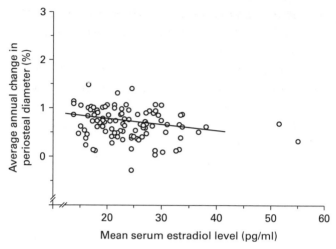

5.7.A Linear association between two normally distributed interval variables

If your scattergram shows that you have a linear relationship between two interval variables, you will want to determine the strength of that relationship. This is done using Pearson's correlation coefficient and/or linear regression.

Pearson's (product-moment) correlation coefficient (also called r) ranges from -1 to $+1$. A correlation of $+1$ indicates that as one variable increases (or decreases) the other variable increases (or decreases) a proportional amount. A correlation of -1 demonstrates an equally strong relationship, but one which goes in the other opposite direction, so as one variable increases (or decreases), the other variable decreases (or increases) in a one-to-one fashion. A correlation of 0 indicates that the two variables have no linear association with one another.

For example, the Pearson's correlation coefficient for the data shown in Figure 5.2 is 0.61, consistent with the strong linear association between the variables. The correlation is positive because higher luminal diameters are associated with larger vasodilator reserve.

In contrast, Ahlborg and colleagues found a weak, negative linear association between mean serum estradiol level and average annual change in periosteal diameter[86] (Figure 5.5). The weak negative association is indicated by the value

---

[86] Ahlborg, H.G., Johnell, O., Turner, C.H., et al. Bone loss and bone size after menopause. *New Engl. J. Med.* 2003; 349: 327–34.

of the Pearson's correlation coefficient of -0.25. The coefficient is negative because higher levels of estradiol are associated with a smaller percentage change in periosteal diameter.

If your correlation is greater than zero, you can test the probability of getting that result by chance assuming there is no association between the two variables. If the probability is very small (<0.05) that the correlation is zero, you can reject the null hypothesis in favor of the hypothesis that there is a linear association between the two variables.

If you square Pearson's correlation coefficient and multiply by 100% ($r^2 \times 100\%$) you get a measure of how much information the two variables share (ranging from 0% to 100%). This can be helpful in gauging the magnitude of an association between two variables, especially with large sample sizes where even a weak linear association may produce a statistically significant P-value.

For example, the Pearson's correlation coefficient for the data shown in Figure 5.2 is statistically significant at a P-value of <0.01, and the two variables "share" about 37% ($0.61^2 \times 100\%$) of information. In contrast, the Pearson's correlation coefficient for the data shown in Figure 5.5 is statistically significant (0.009) although the variables only share 6.25% ($-0.25^2 \times 100$) of their information.

A second method of quantifying a linear association between two variables is to use linear regression.

Least squares linear regression (the most common form of linear regression) determines the line that minimizes the distance between the data points and the line itself.

Unlike Pearson's correlation coefficient, linear regression requires you to "choose" which variable is the independent variable and which one is the dependent variable (outcome). Despite this, remember that linear regression cannot establish causality any more than a correlation coefficient can.

Linear regression yields an equation, which estimates the value of the dependent variable based on an intercept, the coefficient of the independent variable, and the value of the independent variable:

$$\text{outcome} = \text{intercept} + \text{coefficient (independent variable)}$$

The intercept is the point where the regression line crosses the y-axis. The coefficient (also referred to as beta) is the slope of the line. The sign of the coefficient tells you the direction of the line. If the coefficient is positive then the mean value of the outcome increases as the independent variable increases. If the coefficient is negative, then the mean value of the outcome decreases as the independent variable increases.

The size of the slope tells you the steepness of the line. If the slope is 0 then the line is flat: changes in values of the independent variable do not result in any change in the outcome. The larger the absolute value of the slope the steeper the line will be (the larger a change in the mean value of the outcome variable due to a change in the independent variable).

For example, the equation of the line shown in Figure 5.2 is:

coronary vasodilator reserve = 0.47 + 1.3 (minimal luminal diameter)

Use a ruler or the edge of a piece of paper to extend the line shown in Figure 5.2 towards the *y*-axis. Note that the line would intersect the *y*-axis at a point of 0.47.

The coefficient of the independent variable is positive. This is consistent with the observation that as the luminal diameter increases, the coronary vasodilator reserve also increases. In contrast, the coefficient for the independent variable (estradiol level) shown in Figure 5.5 is negative because as estradiol levels increase, changes in periosteal diameter decrease.

The coefficient of the independent variable shown in Figure 5.2 is 1.3. This means that for every millimeter of change of the luminal diameter, the coronary vasodilator reserve will increase by 1.3 units. (A 0.5 mm change would result in a 0.65 unit change in the luminal diameter (1.3 × 0.5 mm) and a 2 mm change would result in a 2.6 unit change in the coronary vasodilator reserve (1.3 × 2.0 mm.))

A potentially misused aspect of linear equation (or any statistical model used for estimating an outcome variable based on an independent variable) is that it allows you to estimate the value of an outcome variable for any value of the independent variable. However, estimating outcomes for values of the independent variable that are not represented (or rarely represented) in your sample is fraught with error. You are essentially in a data free zone. It is for this reason that the authors of Figure 5.5 did not extend the line above 40 pg/ml of estradiol. Although there are two values beyond 40 pg/ml of estradiol, two values are insufficient to be sure that the relationship is linear beyond this point. Similarly, it would have been better if the authors of Figure 5.2 did not extend the line for values above 2.5 mm of luminal diameter, since there is no one with values above this level.

Do not make the same error. Always look at your scatterplot to determine the range of values of your independent variable for which you have enough data to accurately estimate the outcome.

Estimate the outcome variable only for the range of values of your independent variable well represented in your data.

To test the null hypothesis that there is no linear association between the independent variable and the outcome we test the hypothesis that the slope of the line is zero. If the absolute value of the slope is large compared to the standard error associated with it, then the *t*-value associated with the coefficient will be large and the *P*-value will be small. Under these circumstances you can reject the null hypothesis and consider the alternative hypothesis that there is a linear association between the two variables. This method is statistically equivalent to testing the hypothesis that the Pearson's correlation coefficient is zero.

Besides enabling you to estimate the outcome for different values of the independent variable, the other major advantage of linear regression over Pearson's correlation coefficient is that linear regression can be broadened to allow you to assess the impact of multiple variables on outcome (multiple linear regression, Section 6.2).

5.7.B Linear association between two interval variables where at least one is non-normally distributed

> Use Spearman's rank coefficient to test for linear relationships with non-normally distributed interval variables.

When you have an interval variable that is non-normally distributed you cannot use Pearson's correlation coefficient to test for a linear association with another interval variable. Instead, use the Spearman's rank correlation coefficient. This test is the same as the Pearson's correlation coefficient except that the correlation coefficient is based on the rankings of the subjects instead of the actual value of the values of the subjects. In other words, to calculate the Spearman's rank correlation coefficient you first rank the observations separately for each group as I did in Table 5.14 (not together, as I did for calculating the Mann-Whitney test in Table 5.17). Next you use the rankings of the two groups on the variable to calculate the Pearson's correlation coefficient.

For example, in Section 5.6.B, I reviewed a study examining the relationship between coronary inflammation and unstable angina. The investigators measured inflammation using the neutrophil myeloperoxidase index. They found low levels of the index in the coronary vascular circulation, indicating inflammation, in patients with unstable angina. The index does not follow a normal distribution. Therefore, to assess the correlation between the neutrophil myeloperoxidase index and the C-reactive protein level in the blood, a measure of systemic inflammation, they used the Spearman's rank correlation coefficient. The results are shown in Figure 5.6.

From Figure 5.6 there is no way to tell that the correlation is based on the rankings of the subjects rather than their actual scores on these variables. As with Pearson's correlation coefficient, Spearman's rank correlation coefficient does not detect non-linear relationships.

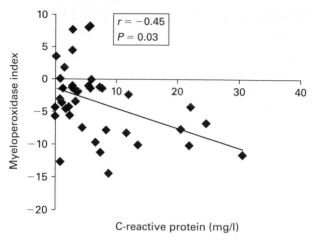

5.8 How do I test an association of two variables when one or both of the variables are ordinal?

> Analyse ordinal variables using non-parametric statistics that are based on rankings.

You will remember that ordinal variables are categorical variables with multiple categories that can be ordered, but for which there is not a fixed interval between the categories, such as stage of cancer (Section 2.10).

Since there is not a fixed interval between the categories, ordinal variables should be analysed by using non-parametric statistics that are based on rankings. As you can see from Table 5.1, many of the tests for ordinal variables are similar to those for non-normally distributed interval variables. Therefore, I will not repeat the explanations in this section. One test for ordinal variables that is important to review is the chi-square for trend. It is not used with interval variables but can be used when you are looking at the association between an ordinal variable and a dichotomous variable (Section 5.8.A).

As the availability of non-parametric statistics is limited, especially if multivariable analysis is needed, investigators will sometimes transform an ordinal variable into a dichotomous variable. This can be done using a natural cut-off, a median split, or comparing extreme categories, just as you would do for a non-normally distributed interval variable (Section 5.4). For example, in a study of health literacy and glycemic (sugar) control among diabetes, health literacy, was measured on an ordinal scale of inadequate, marginal, and adequate.[87] However, the investigators focused only on the two extreme categories (inadequate and adequate literacy). They found that patients with inadequate health literacy were significantly less likely than those with adequate health literacy to have tight glycemic control (OR = 0.51; 95% CI = 0.32–0.79; $P = 0.003$).

At times it may be acceptable to treat an ordinal variable as if it were interval if: (1) there are many categories; and (2) the variable has a normal distribution at each level of the outcome variable and equal variance (Section 5.4); and (3) the sample size is large. However, because the difference between any two levels of an interval scale does not mean the same thing, the interpretation of the results may be difficult.

5.8.A How do I test an association between an ordinal variable and a dichotomous variable (linear trend in proportions)?

The association between an ordinal and a dichotomous variable is tested using chi-squared for trend. The test assesses whether there is an increasing (or decreasing) linear trend in the proportion of subjects at each level of the ordinal variable. The null hypothesis is that there is no linear trend.

For example, Landefeld and colleagues assessed the efficacy of a specialized hospital medical unit in increasing the independence of elderly persons.[88] Persons over the age of 70 years were randomized to an intervention designed to increase the independence or to usual care. The main outcome measure of the study was change in patients' ability to perform basic activities of daily living from admission to discharge. The change was measured on an ordinal scale. The results are shown in Table 5.20.

Comparing the two groups you note that the intervention group is less likely that the usual-care group to be much worse or worse and more likely than the usual-care group to be better or much better. The linear trend is significant at $P = 0.009$.

You might be tempted to perform a standard chi-squared on the data shown in Table 5.19. The problem with treating an ordinal variable as if it were nominal is that you lose the information that the categories are ordered. A standard chi-squared of the above data produces a P-value equal to 0.02. Although the chi-squared is statistically significant when calculated in either way, the chi-squared

[87] Schillinger, D., Grumbach, K., Piette, J., et al. Association of health literacy with diabetes outcomes. *J. Am. Med. Assoc.* 2002; 288: 475–82.
[88] Landefeld, C.S., Palmer, R.M., Kresevic, D.M., Fortinsky, R.H., Kowal, J. A randomized trial of care in a hospital medical unit especially designed to improve the functional outcomes of acutely ill older patients. *New Engl. J. Med.* 1995; 332: 1338–44.

Table 5.20. Functional changes in elders' ability to perform basic activities of daily living

Change from admission to discharge	Intervention group	Usual care
Much worse	26 (9)	25 (8)
Worse	22 (7)	39 (13)
Unchanged	151 (50)	163 (54)
Better	39 (13)	33 (11)
Much better	65 (21)	40 (13)

Values are represented as n (%).

P-value for chi-squared for trend = 0.009.

Data from Landefeld, C.S., et al. A randomized trial of care in a hospital medical unit especially designed to improve the functional outcomes of acutely ill older patients. *New Engl. J. Med.* 1995; 332: 1338–44.

for trend is more informative: it tells you that the intervention is associated with a linear improvement in functional status. The standard chi-squared tells you that the differences in functional status between the intervention group and the usual-care group are unlikely to have occurred by chance.

If your ordinal variable has a large number of levels, such that there are few subjects at some levels, use the Mann-Whitney U-test instead of the chi-squared for trend to evaluate the association (as you would with a non-normally distributed interval variable and a dichotomous variable, Section 5.5.B).

5.9 How do I compare outcomes that occur over time?

In Section 4.6, I reviewed two methods of describing events that occur over time: Kaplan–Meier curves and incident rates based on person-time. These same methods can be used to compare the experience of different groups of patients.

For example, Figure 5.7 shows two Kaplan–Meier curves from a randomized study of patients with acute coronary syndromes.[89] Patients who were randomized to receive blood transfusions were compared on survival to those who were randomized to not receive transfusions. Note that the two curves diverge from one another early and consistently through the follow-up period with patients who received transfusions dying sooner.

In contrast, Figure 5.8 compares the survival of patients randomized to receive coronary artery revascularization to those who were randomized to no

[89] Rao, S.V., Jollis, J.G., Harrington, R.A., et al. Relationship of blood transfusion and clinical outcomes in patients with acute coronary syndromes. *J. Am. Med. Assoc.* 2004; 292: 1555–62.

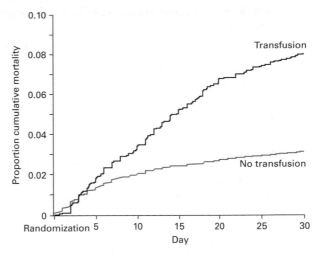

Comparison of survival among patients who received a blood transfusion to those who did not. Reprinted with permission from: Rao, S.V., et al. Relationship of blood transfusion and clinical outcomes in patients with acute coronary syndromes. *J. Am. Med. Assoc.* 2004; 292: 1555–62. Copyright 2004 American Medical Association. All rights reserved.

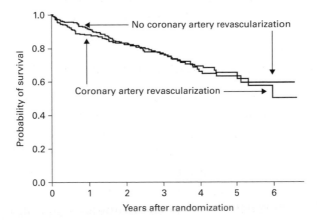

Figure 5.8

Comparison of survival of patients randomized to receive coronary artery revascularization to those who were randomized to no revascularization prior to elective vascular surgery. Reprinted with permission from: McFalls, E.O., et al. Coronary artery revascularization before elective major vascular surgery. *New Engl. J. Med.* 2004; 351: 2795–804. Copyright 1996 Massachusetts Medical Society. All rights reserved.

revascularization prior to elective vascular surgery.[90] As you can see the two Kaplan–Meier curves are essentially superimposed on one another, indicating that coronary artery revascularization does not make a difference.

For Figures 5.7 and 5.8 you do not really need any statistical test to draw the appropriate conclusions. However, most curves are not this obvious, and even when they are, you will still want to present the statistical comparison of the curves.

The most commonly used test to assess the difference between two Kaplan–Meier curves is the log-rank test. We seek to disprove the null hypothesis: that there is no difference in the survival experience of the two groups.

For each time interval, the log-rank test compares the observed number of outcomes in each group to what would have been expected if the two groups had the same survival experience. A time interval is defined by an outcome occurring in either of the groups. The differences between the observed and the expected outcomes for each time interval are then summed. If the difference is large relative to the size of the standard error then the log-rank will be large and the P-value will be small. This is the case with Figure 5.7. The P-value associated with the log-rank test is <0.001. We can therefore reject the null hypothesis and conclude that there is a difference in mortality between persons who received a transfusion and those who did not.

In contrast, if the difference between the groups is small relative to the size of the standard error then the log-rank is small and the P-value is large. This is the case with Figure 5.8. The P-value for the log-rank test is equal to 0.92. We therefore would not reject the null hypothesis that there is no difference in the survival of persons who received coronary artery revascularization compared to those who did not.

Figure 5.9 represents a more complicated situation: the Kaplan–Meier curves cross. Event-free survival is higher among those persons who receive angioplasty initially, but in the latter part of the study (after about 150 days) event-free survival is higher among those who were stented.[91]

Although, the log-rank test is significant ($P = 0.04$) indicating that over the course of the study event-free time is greater with stenting, the log-rank test does not adequately reflect the true complexity of the situation. If you did not review the graphical presentation and went straight to the log-rank test, you would not be able to fully inform your patients that with stenting they are taking on an initially higher risk of an adverse event, but ultimately their chance of avoiding an adverse event is better with a stent. Often when the curves cross, the log-rank

> Use the log-rank test to compare the time to outcome of different groups.

> **Tip**
> Do not rely exclusively on statistical tests to compare survival curves: visually compare them as well.

[90] McFalls, E.O., Ward, H.B., Moritz, T.E., et al. Coronary-artery revascularization before elective major vascular surgery. *New Engl. J. Med.* 2004; 351: 2795–804.

[91] Erbel, R., Haude, M., Hopp, H.W., et al. Coronary-artery stenting compared with balloon angioplasty for restensosis after initial balloon angioplasty. *New Engl. J. Med.* 1998; 339: 1672–8.

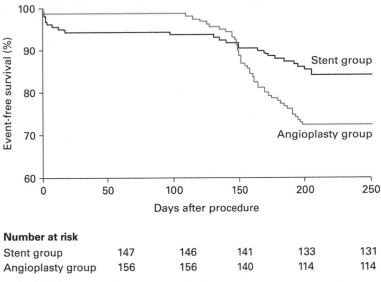

Number at risk					
Stent group	147	146	141	133	131
Angioplasty group	156	156	140	114	114

Figure 5.9   Comparison of event-free survival among patients who received a stent to those who had angioplasty. Reprinted with permission from: Erbel, R., et al. Coronary artery stenting compared with balloon angioplasty for restensosis after initial balloon angioplasty. *New Engl. J. Med.* 1998; 339: 1672–8. Copyright 1996 Massachusetts Medical Society. All rights reserved.

will be non-significant because survival advantages of one group in the beginning of the trial are averaged with survival advantages of the other group at the end of the trial.

The log-rank test is a non-parametric test and therefore does not require that the time to event be normally distributed. In fact, in studies of time to outcome, the data are rarely normally distributed because there are usually a small group of subjects who have substantially longer times to outcome than average.

> The log-rank test does not require that the time to event be normally distributed.

The log-rank test can also be used to compare time to outcome for more than two groups. In such cases you are testing the null hypothesis that the survival experience does not significantly differ among the groups.

As with performing a chi-squared test or ANOVA with more than two groups, a significant log-rank does not tell you where the difference lies. To determine this you can perform pairwise comparisons of the curves. But to avoid capitalizing on chance, set a more stringent standard (i.e., a lower *P*-value) before concluding that differences are not due to chance. You can do this by using the Bonferroni correction (Section 5.6.A). For example, if you are performing all possible pairwise comparisons of three curves – three – than you would set the threshold for disproving the null hypothesis of 0.017 (0.05/3).

Table 5.21. Incidence of pneumonia with and without exposure to acid-suppressive drugs

	Exposed to acid suppressive drugs	Unexposed
Person-years of observation	7562	970,331
Number of cases of pneumonia	185	5366
Incidence rate of pneumonia per 100 person-years	2.45	0.55

Data from Laheij, R.J.F., et al. Risk of community-acquired pneumonia and use of gastric acid-suppressive drugs. *J. Am. Med. Assoc.* 2004; 292: 1955–60.

Some investigators use the Wilcoxon test[92] (also known as Geham's test) to compare the survival experience of different groups of subjects. The Wilcoxon test weighs outcomes that occur early in the study more heavily than outcomes that occur later on. For this reason, if there is a large difference between the groups in the number of early outcomes you may find that the Wilcoxon test is statistically significant while the log-rank test is not. However, generally we weigh early and late outcomes about equally and for this reason you will rarely see the Wilcoxon test used.

5.9.A Incident rates for comparison of two groups

We can also use incidence rates to compare two groups. For example, Laheij and colleagues compared the incidence of community-acquired pneumonia among patients exposed to acid suppressing drugs and those who are unexposed (Table 5.21).[93] (The impetus for this study is the thought that stomach acid is protective against pneumonia because the acid kills bacteria.)

The incidence of pneumonia in patients exposed to acid suppressing drugs is 2.45 per 100 person years ($185/7562 \times 100$) and the incidence of pneumonia in unexposed patients is 0.55 per 100 person years ($5366/970,331 \times 100$) (Table 5.21). You can compute a z-statistic to calculate whether the incidence rates are statistically different. The formula for the z-statistic is readily available and can be calculated by hand.[94] In this case, the difference was statistically significant at the P level < 0.001.

---

[92] The Wilcoxon test is not the same as the Wilcoxon rank sum test (Section 5.5.B) or the Wilcoxon signed rank test (Section 5.10).

[93] Laheij, R.J.F., Sturkenboom, M.C.J.M., Hassing, R., Dieleman, J., Stricker, B.H.C., Jansen, J.B.M.J. Risk of community-acquired pneumonia and use of gastric acid-suppressive drugs. *J. Am. Med. Assoc.* 2004; 292: 1955–60.

[94] Rosner, B. *Fundamentals of Biostatistics* (5th edition). California: Duxbury, 2000, pp. 684–5.

More commonly, the difference between two measures of incidence is assessed using the rate ratio (also known as the incidence density ratio). The rate ratio equals:

$$\text{rate ratio} = \frac{\text{incidence rate for exposed}}{\text{incidence rate for unexposed}}$$

In the case of the data shown in Table 5.21, the rate ratio is:

$$\text{rate ratio} = \frac{2.45}{0.55} = 4.5$$

As with risk ratios or odds ratios, rate ratios should be reported with 95% confidence intervals. In the case of this study the 95% confidence intervals are 3.8–5.1.

5.10 How do I analyse repeated observations of the same subject?

A common clinical research design involves observing the same subjects on multiple occasions (e.g., at 6-month intervals) or under different conditions (e.g., before or after treatment).

Repeated observations of the same subject may occur due to multiple observations over time or due to subjects receiving different types of treatments.

In either case, we have repeated measurements of the same subjects. In the simplest cases we are evaluating differences in the repeated measurements of a single sample of subjects. In more complex models we are comparing changes in the repeated measurements of two or more samples of subjects.

> Repeated observations of the same subject must be analysed with statistics that take into account that the observations are correlated.

The bivariate statistics that we have reviewed so far assume that the observations are independent of one another. This is not the case with repeated observations of the same subjects. The observations are not independent of one another because the *same* subject is more likely to respond in a similar way at a repeat examination or under a different condition than a different subject. Repeated observations of the same subject must be analysed with statistics that take into account that the repeated observations are correlated.[95]

---

[95] The analysis of correlated outcome data is a complicated issue. Besides repeated observations of the same individuals, there are other circumstances that lead to correlated outcomes including matched studies (Section 5.11), clustered study designs where subjects have been recruited from multiple settings of related individuals (e.g., families, doctor's practices, or hospitals) and observations of different body parts of the same person. Analysis of correlated outcome data often requires multivariable modeling. Readers who want to know more about this important area of clinical research should see: Katz, M.H. *Multivariable Analysis: A Practical Guide for Clinicians* (2nd edition). Cambridge University Press, 2005, pp. 158–78.

Table 5.22. Comparison of bivariate tests for independent observations and repeated observations of the same subjects.

	Independent observations (2 groups)	Paired observations (2 observations)	Independent observations (≥3 groups)	Repeated observations (≥3 observations)
Dichotomous variable	Chi-squared Fisher's exact	McNemar's test	Chi-squared	Cochran's Q
Normally distributed interval variable	t-test	Paired t-test	ANOVA	Repeated-measures ANOVA
Non-normally distributed interval variable	Mann-Whitney test	Wilcoxon signed rank test	Kruskal–Wallis test	Friedman statistic
Ordinal variable	Mann-Whitney test	Wilcoxon signed rank test	Kruskal–Wallis test	Friedman statistic

If you do not take into account the correlation of repeated observations, your results will be inaccurate. The most common effect is to exaggerate the statistical significance of your results. To understand why consider that you wish to assess whether men or women have higher cholesterol levels. Which would provide you with more information: the cholesterol results of 200 subjects (100 men and 100 women) or the cholesterol results of 50 subjects (25 men and 25 women) taken four times? The answer is the former because subjects would be expected to have similar cholesterol results each time their level is checked. Therefore, you do not learn as much from having three additional readings as having an additional 150 subjects undergo cholesterol testing.

A comparison of bivariate tests for independent observations and repeated observations are shown in Table 5.22. When there are only two repeated observations they are often referred to as paired observations.

5.10.A Paired measurements of a dichotomous variable

Use McNemar's test to assess paired observations on a dichotomous outcome.

When you have paired observations (i.e., before and after) of a dichotomous variable use McNemar's test.

For example, Kuipers and colleagues sought to determine the likelihood that long-term acid suppression would result in gastritis.[96] They followed 59 patients with gastroesophageal reflux disease and *Heliobacter pylori*. All patients were treated with an acid suppresser (omeprazole); the average duration of treatment was 5 years.

---

[96] Kuipers, E.J., Lundell, L., Klinkenberg-Knol, E.C., et al. Atrophic gastritis and *Helicobacter pylori* infection in patients with reflux esophagitis treated with omeprazole or fundoplication. *New Engl. J. Med.* 1996; 334: 1018–22.

Table 5.23. Presence of gastritis among patients with gastroesophageal reflux and *H. pylori* infection

Baseline	Follow-up		Total
	Normal	Gastritis	
Normal	7	**17**	24 (41%)
Gastritis	**4**	31	35 (59%)
Total	11 (19%)	48 (81%)	59 (100%)

$P = 0.007$ by McNemar's test.
Data from Kuipers, E.J., et al. Atrophic gastritis and *Helicobacter pylori* in patients with reflux esophagitis treated with omeprazole or fundoplication. *New Engl. J. Med.* 1996; 334: 1018–22.

At baseline 41% of patients had normal mucosa and 59% had gastritis (Table 5.23, last column) while at follow-up only 19% had normal mucosa and 81% had gastritis (bottom row).

For calculating McNemar's test the only two cells that matter are the two cells that indicate change (i.e., going from normal at baseline to having gastritis at follow-up or going from gastritis at baseline to having a normal examination at follow-up). I have bolded these two cells in Table 5.23. Adding these two cells together, we find that 21 patients had a change in status. If there were no tendency toward gastritis in patients with gastroesophageal reflux we would expect that about half of these 21 patients (10.5 patients) would go in each direction (half from normal to gastritis and half from gastritis to normal).

However, our distribution (4 and 17) is clearly different from 10.5. Is it possible that the difference is due to chance? We use McNemar's test to determine the probability of obtaining these results if the null hypothesis (no difference) were true. In the case of this example, the probability is equal to 0.007. We can therefore reject the null hypothesis and consider alternative hypotheses, such as long-term acid suppression leads to the development of gastritis.

To appreciate the importance of using an analytic tool that incorporates the pairing of observations, let us assume that you analysed the data shown in Table 5.23 as if the observations were unpaired. Feeling smart from having read Section 5.2 you bypass chi-squared because you recognize that the expected number of subjects in one of the cells (normal at baseline and normal at follow-up) is <5 ($0.41 \times 11 = 4.5$). The *P*-value associated with a two-tailed Fisher's exact test is 0.10. Therefore, you would wrongly assume that the null hypothesis is correct: that there is no significant difference between the baseline and the follow-up examination.

Table 5.24. Changes in behaviors associated with HIV transmission*

	Baseline (%)	6 months (%)	12 months (%)	18 months (%)	P-value
HIV-positive sex partner	20	18	18	10	<0.001
Unprotected receptive anal sex	32	27	28	29	0.02
Condom failure	19	13	10	12	<0.001
Urethritis	9	3	2	2	<0.001

* Behaviors are coded as yes or no.

Data from Buchbinder, S.P., et al. Feasibility of human immunodeficiency virus vaccine trials in homosexual men in the United States: risk behavior, seroincidence, and willingness to participate. *J. Infect. Dis.* 1996; 174: 954–61.

5.10.B Three or more repeated measurements of a dichotomous variable

> Use Cochran's Q to assess multiple observations of a dichotomous variable on the same subjects.

When you have multiple observations of a dichotomous variable on the same subjects use Cochran's Q.

Cochran's Q follows a chi-squared distribution. When the value is large you can reject the null hypothesis that there are no differences among the repeated observations of the subjects.[97]

For example, Buchbinder and colleagues analysed changes in behaviors associated with HIV transmission among 1256 HIV-negative men who have sex with men.[98] Subjects were assessed at baseline, at 6, 12, and 18 months. The investigators compared the percent of subjects engaging in each behavior at the four different times by calculating Cochran's Q-test for each of the four behaviors. In other words, they calculated four Cochran's Q-tests, each of which has a P-value, as shown in Table 5.24. They found that there were significant differences in the percentages of subjects engaging in the four behaviors over time.

5.10.C Paired measurements of a normally distributed interval variable

> Use a paired t-test to compare paired observations of a normally distributed interval variable.

When you have a paired observation of a normally distributed interval variable use the paired t-test.

The paired t-test for repeated observations is calculated as the mean change between the paired observations divided by the standard deviation of that change.

$$\text{paired } t = \frac{\text{mean change in the pair}}{\text{standard deviation of the change}}$$

---

[97] For more on Cochran's Q.: Fleiss, J.L., Levin, B., Paik, M.C. *Statistical Methods for Rates and Proportions* (3rd edition). Hoboken, New Jersey: Wiley & Sons, 2003, pp. 126–33.

[98] Buchbinder, S.P., Douglas, J.M., McKirnan, D.J., et al. Feasibility of human immunodeficiency virus vaccine trials in homosexual men in the United States: risk behavior, seroincidence, and willingness to participate. *J. Infect. Dis.* 1996: 174: 954–61.

Table 5.25. Effect of cocaine use, cigarettes, and cocaine plus cigarettes on coronary artery stenosis

Exposure	Pre-exposure stenosis diameter (mm)	Post-exposure stenosis diameter (mm)	P-value*
Cocaine use ($n = 6$)	1.21	1.09	0.01
Cigarette ($n = 12$)	1.13	1.07	0.32
Cocaine plus cigarette ($n = 12$)	1.20	0.96	<0.001

*P-value based on a paired *t*-test.

Data from Moliterno, D.J., Willard, J.E., Lange, R.A., et al. Coronary-artery vasoconstriction induced by cocaine, cigarette smoking, or both. *New Engl. J. Med.* 1994; 330: 454–9.

As with the unpaired *t*-test, large *t*-values are associated with small *P*-values. When the *P*-value is small the likelihood that the observed difference is due to chance is low.

For example, Moliterno and colleagues assessed the effect of cocaine and cigarette smoking on coronary artery vasoconstriction.[99] They compared the degree of coronary artery stenosis (measured using coronary angiography) before and after three different exposures received by three different groups of subjects. One group ($n = 6$) were exposed to intranasal cocaine use. A second group ($n = 12$) was exposed to cigarette smoke; a third group was exposed to both intranasal cocaine use and cigarette smoke. For each group, the investigators used a paired *t*-test to compare the diameter of the stenosis at baseline to the diameter following exposure.

In all three groups there was a narrowing of the stenosis (vasoconstriction); the narrowing was statistically significant (as indicated by the *P*-value of the paired *t*-test) with cocaine use and with cocaine use plus smoking (Table 5.25).

5.10.D Multiple ($\geq$3) repeated observations of a normally distributed interval variable

> Use repeated-measures ANOVA to assess repeated observations of a normally distributed interval variable.

When you have repeated observations of a normally distributed interval variable use repeated-measures ANOVA.

The simplest type of repeated-measures ANOVA is the comparison of the response of a single group of subjects on three or more occasions. It is analogous to a paired *t*-test (Section 5.10.C) except you have more than two measurements.

---

[99] Moliterno, D.J., Willard, J.E., Lange, R.A., et al. Coronary artery vasoconstriction induced by cocaine, cigarette smoking, or both. *New Engl. J. Med.* 1994; 330: 454–9.

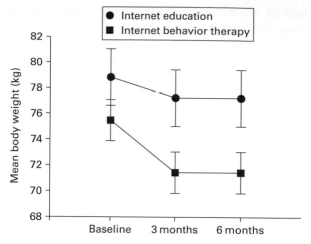

Comparison of weight loss among participants receiving internet education to those who received internet behavioral therapy. Reprinted with permission from: Tate, D.F., et al. Using internet technology to deliver a behavioral weight loss program. *J. Am. Med. Assoc.* 2001; 285: 1172–7. Copyright 2001 American Medical Association. All rights reserved.

As with standard ANOVA (Section 5.6.A) repeated-measures ANOVA produces an *F*-value. If the value of *F* is large, and the *P*-value is small, you can reject the null hypothesis (that the means of the different observations are the same).

Repeated-measures ANOVA can also be used to compare repeated observations of two or more groups of subjects. In this case, we are testing the null hypothesis that the repeated means are not different between the groups. If the value of *F* is large, and the *P*-value is small, we can reject the null hypothesis.

For example, Tate and colleagues compared two behavioral weight loss programs.[100] Participants were randomized to receive either education or behavioral therapy (both over the internet!). Weight was assessed at baseline, 3 months, and 6 months. The null hypothesis was that there was no difference in the measured weight of the two groups over time.

As you can see in Figure 5.10 participants who received the behavioral therapy had greater weight loss over time than those that received the education. Repeated-measures ANOVA indicated that the difference in weight loss between the two groups over time was significant at $P = 0.005$.

Unfortunately, repeated-measures ANOVA has several limitations. Specifically, you must have the same number of observations of each subject and the observations must be made at the same time. Since these conditions are not

[100] Tate, D.F., Wing, R.R., Winett, R.A. Using internet technology to deliver a behavioral weight loss program. *J. Am. Med. Assoc.* 2001; 285: 1172–7.

usually met with clinical studies, investigators more commonly use generalized estimating equations or mixed-effects models in these situations. These techniques are beyond the scope of this book.[101]

5.10.E Paired observations of a non-normally distributed interval variable or an ordinal variable

> Use the Wilcoxon signed rank test to compare paired observations of a non-normally distributed interval variable or of an ordinal variable.

When you have paired observations of a non-normally distributed interval variable or of an ordinal variable use the Wilcoxon signed rank test (also known as the Wilcoxon matched pairs test).

The test is based on ranking the differences between the paired observations. Specifically, for each pair of observations, you can calculate a difference. In some cases that difference will be positive (if the first observation is higher than second observation). In other cases that difference will be negative (if the first observation is lower than the second observation). If a similar numbers of pairs have positive rankings as negative rankings, then when you add up the ranks you will get zero (or a value close to zero). If the rankings are overwhelmingly positive or negative, then when you add up the rankings, you will get a large absolute number. (An absolute number is the number without consideration of a positive or negative sign.)

If the absolute value is large for a given sample size, then the P-value will be small and you can reject the null hypothesis that there is no difference between the two sets of observations.

For example, Davi and colleagues compared the urinary 11-dehydro-thromboxane B_2 excretion levels among 11 obese women before and after weight loss.[102] (11-dehydro-thromboxane B_2 is a marker of platelet activation; platelet activation may be one of the intervening factors between obesity and increased risk of cardiovascular disease.) You can see from Figure 5.11 that the level of 11-dehydro-thromboxane B_2 declined in the vast majority of women.

Although the urinary 11-dehydro-thromboxane B_2 excretion levels are measured on an interval scale, the distribution was skewed. With a skewed distribution and a small sample size, a paired t-test would not be valid. Instead, the authors used a Wilcoxon signed rank test and found that there was a statistically significant ($P < 0.05$) decrease in urinary 11-dehydro-thromboxane B_2 excretion levels from after weight loss.

---

[101] Katz, M.H. *Multivariable Analysis: A Practical Guide for Clinicians* (2nd edition). Cambridge University Press, 2005, Chapter 12.
[102] Davi, G., Guagnana, M.T., Ciabattoni, G., et al. Platelet activation in obese women: role of inflammation and oxidant stress. *J. Am. Med. Assoc.* 2002; 288: 2008–14.

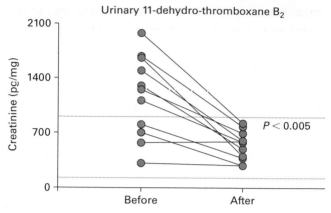

Urinary 11-dehydro-thromboxane B$_2$ excretion levels among 11 obese women before and after weight loss. The dotted lines indicate the range of excretion of 11-dehydro-thromboxane B$_2$ excretion levels among non-obese women. Reprinted with permission from Davi, G., et al. Platelet activation in obese women: role of inflammation and oxidant stress. *J. Am. Med. Assoc.* 2002; 288: 2008–14. Copyright 2002 American Medical Association. All rights reserved.

Herrstedt and colleagues used the Wilcoxon signed rank test to compare paired observations of an ordinal variable.[103] The ordinal variable was severity of nausea and the study was a randomized, double-blinded crossover trial of two different antiemetic regimens: ondansetron or ondansetron plus metopimazine. All patients were receiving chemotherapy. Each patient received one regimen on a round of chemotherapy and the other regimen on the next round of chemotherapy.

Patients who received ondansetron plus metopimazine were more likely to have no or mild nausea and more less likely to have moderate or severe nausea than patients who received only ondansetron (Table 5.26). The Wilcoxon signed rank test was significant ($P = 0.006$).

5.10.F Repeated (≥3) observations of a non-normally distributed interval variable or an ordinal variable

> Use the Friedman statistic to assess repeated observations of a non-normally distributed interval variable or an ordinal variable.

When you have repeated observations of a non-normally distributed interval variable or an ordinal variable use the Friedman statistic.

The Friedman statistic, like the Wilcoxon signed rank test, is based on rankings. The test ranks the multiple observations of each subject, sums the rankings

[103] Herrstedt, J., Sigsgaard, T., Boesgaard, M., Jensen, T.P., Dombernowsky, P. Ondansetron plus metopimazine compared with ondansetron alone in patients receiving moderately emetogenic chemotherapy. *New Engl. J. Med.* 1993; 328: 1076–80.

Table 5.26. Response of 30 chemotherapy patients to two different regimens

	Antiemetic regimen	
Severity of nausea	Ondansetron	Ondansetron + metopimazine
None	6 (20)	12 (40)
Mild	9 (30)	10 (33)
Moderate	10 (33)	8 (27)
Severe	5 (17)	0 (0)

Values are represented as n (%).

P-value of Wilcoxon signed rank test = 0.006.

Data from Herrstedt, J., et al. Ondansetron plus metopimazine compared with ondansetron alone in patients receiving moderately emetogenic chemotherapy. *New Engl. J. Med.* 1993; 328: 1076–80.

under each condition (or time point) and compares the observed rank sums for each condition to what would be expected by chance.

What you would expect by chance is that the observed rank sums for the different conditions would be about the same. However, if the rankings come out substantially higher (or lower) for one of the conditions, then the Friedman statistic will yield a small P-value and you can reject the null hypothesis that there are no differences in the observations at the different conditions/time points.

For example, Darzins and colleagues assessed differences in the type of care subjects preferred depending on whether the care was for an unfamiliar person, a family member, or for himself or herself.[104] The type of care was an interval scale range from palliative care to intensive care. The sample included doctors, nurses, health professionals, high school students and members of the general public. Respondents were given a clinical vignette about an 82-year-old-man with dementia who arrives in the emergency department with life-threatening gastrointestinal bleeding. No guidance on the type of care that the patient would want is available from the patient or his family. The respondent is asked to say how the patient should be treated under three different conditions: that the vignette patient is unfamiliar to the subject, that the patient is a family member of the subject, or that the subject is the patient, himself or herself.

There were dramatic differences in the subjects' choice of care depending on whether they were choosing it for an unfamiliar person, a family member,

---

[104] Darzins, R., Molloy, D.W., Harrison, C. Treatment for life-threatening illness. *New Engl. J. Med.* 1993; 329: 736.

Table 5.27. Choice of type of care for life-threatening condition in a patient with dementia

Type of care	Unfamiliar patient (%)	Family member (%)	Self (%)
Palliative	37	54	68
Limited	39	31	23
Surgical	12	8	4
Intensive	13	7	5

Friedman statistic is significant, $P < 0.001$. Data from Darzins, R., et al. Treatment for life-threatening illness. *New Engl. J. Med.* 1993; 329: 736

or for themselves (Table 5.27). The Friedman statistic was significant at $P < 0.001$.[105]

5.11 How do I test bivariate associations with matched data?

Matching is a useful strategy for eliminating confounding, especially for small case–control studies (Section 2.6.C). However, when you individually match cases and controls you need to use an analytic method that incorporates the matching. Table 5.28 compares tests used to assess associations with unmatched and matched data (two groups).

As I hope you notice, most of the tests for matched data shown in Table 5.28 are the same as the tests for paired observations of the same subject shown in Table 5.22. That's because repeated observations of the same subject are essentially matched analyses where the subject is serving as his or her own control.

5.11.A Matched comparisons of a dichotomous variable

Use McNemar's test to compare matched data on a dichotomous outcome.

When you wish to compare the matched pairs on a dichotomous variable use McNemar's test (just as you would with paired observations of the same person on a dichotomous variable, Section 5.10.A).

Just as when using McNemar's test with paired observations only the discordant pairs contribute to the determination of McNemar's test.

---

[105] As this study asks subjects to make hypothetical decisions you may feel that it does not qualify as repeated "observations" of the same subjects. But it is repeated decision-making by subjects under different hypothetical conditions.

Table 5.28. Comparison of bivariate tests for unmatched and matched data

	Unmatched data	Matched data
Dichotomous variable	Chi-squared	McNemar's test
	Odds ratio	Matched odds ratio
Normally distributed interval variable	t-test	Paired t-test
Non-normally distributed variable	Mann-Whitney test	Wilcoxon signed rank test
Ordinal variable	Mann-Whitney test	Wilcoxon signed rank test
Survival time	Log-rank	No readily available test

For example, Kujala and colleagues compared the mortality of twin pairs due to smoking.[106] There were 84 twin pairs that were discordant on both the risk factor (one twin smoked and one twin did not smoke) and the outcome (one twin died and one did not). If smoking were unrelated to mortality then we would expect that for half of the pairs it would be the smoker who died and for the other half it would be the nonsmoking twin who died. In fact, in 67 of the pairs it was the smoker in the pair who died, and in only 17 of the pairs was it the nonsmoker who died. McNemar's test was significant at $P < 0.001$.

Besides McNemar's test, the matched odds ratio is often used to report the results for matched studies. It is easy to compute. It is:

$$\text{matched odds ratio} = \frac{\text{number of pairs where the one with the risk factor experiences the outcome}}{\text{number of pairs where the one without the risk factor experiences the outcome}}$$

In the case of Kujala and colleagues study of smoking and mortality among twins, the matched odds ratio is:

$$\frac{67}{17} = 3.9$$

---

[106] Kujala, U.M., Kaprio, J., Koskenvuo, M. Modifiable risk factors as predictors of all-cause mortality: the roles of genetics and childhood environment. *Am. J. Epidemiol.* 2002; 156: 985–93.

Table 5.29. Comparison of sleep characteristics of 1st-degree relatives with sleep apnea/hypopnea compared to controls

	Cases* (mean)	Controls (mean)	P-value[†]
Slow wave (deep) sleep	78 min	91 min	0.03
Minutes of light sleep	209 min	179 min	0.006
2% desaturations	6/h	3/h	0.04
3% desaturations	4/h	2/h	0.04

*Cases are 1st-degree relatives of patients with sleep apnea.
[†]P-value is based on paired t-test.
Data from Mathur, R. and Douglas, N.J. Family studies in patients with the sleep apnea–hyponea syndrome. *Ann. Intern. Med.* 1995; 122: 174–8.

5.11.B Matched measurements of a normally distributed interval variable

When you have matched data on a normally distributed interval variable use a paired t-test (just as you would with paired measures of the same person on a normally distributed interval variable, Section 5.10.C).

For example, Mathur and colleagues conducted a case–control study of whether familial factors were associated with development of sleep apnea/hypopnea.[107] The investigators matched 51 1st-degree relatives of patients with sleep apnea (cases) to 51 controls of similar age, sex, height, and weight. They used paired t-tests to compare cases to their matched controls on several normally distributed interval variables.

The paired t-test for comparing matched results is the same as the paired t-test for comparing two measurements of the same person. The only difference is that with the former the "pair" is the case and the control and with the latter the pair is the two measurements.

As you can see, 1st-degree relatives had significantly less slow wave (deep) sleep, more light sleep, and more 2% and 3% oxyhemoglobin desaturations per hour than controls (Table 5.29).

5.11.C Matched measurements of a non-normally distributed interval or ordinal variable

When you have matched data on a non-normally distributed interval or ordinal variable use the Wilcoxon signed rank test (just as you would with

---

[107] Mathur, R., Douglas, N.J. Family studies in patients with the sleep apnea–hypopnea syndrome. *Ann. Intern. Med.* 1995; 122: 174–8.

Table 5.30. Comparison of sleep characteristics of 1st-degree relatives with sleep apnea/hypopnea to controls

	Cases (median)	Controls (median)	P-value[†]
Apnea plus hyponea frequency	13/h	4/h	<0.001
Arousals per hour	30/h	17/h	<0.001

*Cases are 1st-degree relatives of patients with sleep apnea.

[†]P-value is based on Wilcoxon signed rank test.

Data from Mathur, R., and Douglas, N.J. Family studies in patients with the sleep apnea-hyponea syndrome. *Ann. Intern. Med.* 1995; 122: 174–8.

paired measurements of the same subject on a non-normally distributed interval or ordinal variable, Section 5.10.E).

For example, in the same sleep apnea study discussed above the investigators compared cases and controls on two non-normally distributed interval variables. They found, using the Wilcoxon signed rank test, that cases had significantly higher apnea–hypnoea frequency and more arousals per hour (Table 5.30).

Taken together, the data shown in Tables 5.29 and 5.30 suggest that there is a strong familial component to the sleep apnea–hypopnea syndrome.

5.11.D Matched survival time

Survival analysis cannot incorporate matched observations.

For survival analyses there are no readily available statistical techniques that incorporate matching. Therefore, you would need to "abandon" the matching, and analyse your data as if they were unmatched. Although the individual matching will not be incorporated in the analysis, matching still helps to assure that your controls and cases are comparable.

Multivariable statistics

6.1 What is multivariable analysis? Why is it necessary?

Multivariable analysis is a statistical tool for determining the unique (independent) contributions of various factors to a single event or outcome.

A risk factor is independently associated with an outcome when the effect persists after taking into account the other risk factors and confounders.

Multivariable analysis is a statistical tool for determining the unique (independent) contributions of various factors to a single event or outcome.[108] It is an essential tool because most clinical events have more than one cause and a number of potential confounders.

For example, we know from bivariate analysis that cigarette smoking, obesity, a sedentary life style, hypertension, and diabetes are associated with an increased risk for coronary artery disease.

But are these risk factors *independent* of one another? By independent, we mean, that the risk factor predicts the outcome even after taking the other risk factors into account. Conversely, is it possible that these risk factors only appear to be related to coronary artery disease because the relationship between the risk factor and the outcome is confounded by a third factor. Perhaps the only reason that lack of exercise is associated with decreased coronary artery disease is that smokers exercise less and because they exercise less they become obese, and their obesity leads to higher blood pressure and greater insulin resistance.

The question of whether a risk factor is independently associated with an outcome is of more than academic significance. For example, if the association of exercise and coronary artery disease is confounded by smoking, then encouraging people to exercise more will not change their risk of coronary artery disease.

Conversely if the impact of exercise on coronary artery disease is independent of smoking status, then exercising more will lower the risk of coronary artery disease even if the person continues to smoke. In fact, a number of multivariable analyses have demonstrated that lack of exercise is independently associated with coronary artery disease.

---

[108] It is impossible to do justice to multivariable analysis in a single chapter. That's why I wrote a book on it: Katz, M.H. *Multivariable Analysis: A Practical Guide for Clinicians* (2nd edition). New York: Cambridge University Press, 2005. This chapter draws heavily from that book and from Katz, M.H. Multivariable analysis: a primer for readers of medical research. *Ann. Intern. Med.* 2003; 138: 644–50.

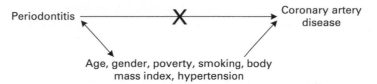

Figure 6.1   Periodontitis is not associated with coronary artery disease after adjustment for confounders.

Let's consider another example. Is periodontitis (an inflammation of the gums with breakdown of the surrounding bone) independently associated with coronary heart disease? An increase in the risk of a myocardial infarction due to periodontitis is biologically plausible: periodontitis results in chronic low-level bacteremia and an elevation of inflammatory mediators, either of which could result in increased coronary heart disease.

Hujoel and colleagues used a prospective cohort design to evaluate whether periodontitis is independently associated with coronary heart disease. Consistent with prior studies, bivariate analysis demonstrated that persons with periodontitis had a markedly increased rate of coronary heart disease (relative hazard (RH) = 2.66; 95% CI = 2.34–3.03).[109] If this relationship were independent and causal, then interventions that reduced periodontitis would decrease the occurrence of coronary heart disease.

The investigators used multivariable analysis to adjust for a number of potential confounders including older age, male sex, poverty, smoking, higher body mass index, and hypertension. With these variables in the model, along with a statistical adjustment for sampling design and sampling weights, they found that the association between periodontitis and coronary heart disease weakened substantially: the hazard ratio decreased to 1.21; the 95% confidence intervals for the hazard ratio (RH = 0.98–1.50) included one; and the association between periodontitis and coronary artery disease was no longer statistically significant.

In other words, as shown in Figure 6.1, periodontitis is not independently associated with coronary heart disease; the apparent association is due to confounding by other factors. Treating periodontitis will not decrease the risk of coronary heart disease – at least not according to this study – although it will decrease the risk of losing your teeth!

Multivariable analysis is not the only method of eliminating confounding. In the design phase of your study you can eliminate confounding through randomization and matching (Sections 2.3.A and 2.6.C). However, these strategies cannot

| Matching and randomization are used to minimize confounding in the design phase of a study. |

[109] Hujoel, P.P., Drangsholt, M., Spiekerman, C., DeRouen, T.A. Periodontal disease and coronary heart disease risk. *J. Am. Med. Assoc.* 2000; 284: 1406–10.

be used once your data are collected. In addition, both strategies have limitations that may make them undesirable for your study. For example, there are so many factors known to be causally related to coronary heart disease that it would be very cumbersome to assemble your samples if you needed to match for all these characteristics. Moreover, randomization will not work for many of these characteristics because subjects cannot be randomized to them (e.g., smoking, hypertension, etc.).

In the analysis phase, besides multivariable analysis, you can use stratification to eliminate confounding. For example, the impact of smoking on coronary heart disease can be examined separately for males and females, thereby eliminating the possibility that sex confounds the relationship between smoking and coronary heart disease. If smoking is significantly associated with coronary heart disease among both men and women – as is the case – then we can say that the impact of smoking on coronary artery disease is independent of sex.

Stratification works well in situations where there are no more than one or two confounders. However, to determine the independent relationship of smoking and coronary artery disease you would need to stratify not only for sex, but also for those other factors known to be associated with smoking and causally related to coronary artery disease, including obesity, hypertension, and sedentary life style. This would create a large and unwieldy number of subgroups in which you would need to determine the relationship between the risk factor and the outcome. As the sample sizes of the subgroups would be small, the estimates of risk would be unstable.

The strength of multivariable analysis is that it enables us to statistically adjust for many potential confounders. Using multivariable analysis we can demonstrate that after adjusting for male sex, obesity, hypertension, and sedentary life style, smoking has an *independent* relationship with coronary artery disease (Figure 6.2).

Even in situations where there should be no confounding, such as in randomized controlled trials, multivariable analysis is often used. There are several reasons for this. First, even though randomization should result in groups equal with respect to both known and unknown factors, randomization can sometimes, by chance, result in one group being significantly different from another on a particular variable. Adjusting for this variable will lessen concerns that your results are confounded by that variable. Further, with certain types of multivariable analysis, the unadjusted estimate of the exposure may not be correct if the impact of the risk factor on the outcome varies across the different groups of subjects.[110] Finally, for better or for worse, multivariable analysis has become the standard for showing that confounding is not affecting the results.

> Multivariable analysis and stratification are used to minimize confounding in the analytic phase of a study.

> Stratification works well in minimizing confounding in situations where there are no more than one or two confounders.

---

[110] Harrell, F.E. *Regression Modeling Strategies*. New York: Springer, 2001, p. 4.

Table 6.1. Type of outcome variable determines choice of multivariable analysis

Type of outcome	Example of outcome variable	Type of multivariable analysis
Interval	Blood pressure, weight, temperature	Multiple linear regression
Dichotomous	Death, cancer, intensive care unit admission	Multiple logistic regression
Time to outcome (dichotomous event)	Time to death, time to cancer	Proportional hazards analysis

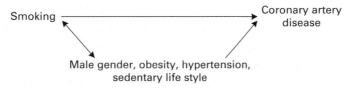

Figure 6.2   Smoking is associated with coronary artery disease even after adjustment for confounders.

6.2 How do I choose what type of multivariable analysis to use?

Three types of multivariable analysis are used commonly in clinical research: multiple linear regression, multiple logistic regression, and proportional hazards (Cox) analysis.[111]

The major determinant of the type of multivariable analysis to use is the nature of the outcome variable (Table 6.1). Multiple linear regression is used with interval outcomes (e.g., blood pressure). Multiple logistic regression is used with dichotomous outcomes (e.g., death (yes/no)). Proportional hazards analysis (a type of survival analysis) is used with length of time to a dichotomous outcome (e.g., time from baseline visit to death).

6.3 What should I do if my outcome variable is ordinal or nominal?

Ordinal (multiple categories that can be ordered) and nominal (multiple categories that cannot be ordered) outcomes (Section 2.10) are harder to study using multivariable analysis. For this reason, the most common way of treating ordinal and nominal outcomes in multivariable analysis is to dichotomize them.

---

[111] Other important multivariable techniques include analysis of variance (for interval outcomes) and Poisson regression (for rare outcomes and counts) see: Katz, M.H. *Multivariable Analysis: A Practical Guide for Clinicians* (2nd edition). New York: Cambridge University Press, 2005.

For example, the ordinal variable New York Heart Association Classification (Section 2.10) is often grouped as levels I and II (no or mild limitation in exercise tolerance) versus levels III and IV (moderate or severe limitation in exercise tolerance). Similarly, the nominal variable, cause of death, may be classified as cardiovascular disease: yes or no. Obviously, such groupings result in loss of information.

Alternatively, the data can be analysed using an adaptation of logistic regression. Ordinal outcomes can be analysed using proportional odds logistic regression and nominal outcomes can be analysed using polytomous logistic regression. As these techniques are not commonly used in medical research, they will not be described here, but readers can obtain more information about these methods from other sources.[112] Another technique available for nominal outcomes is discriminant function analysis. It has both similarities to and differences from the three major methods described here.[113]

> Ordinal and nominal outcomes can be analysed using adaptations of logistic regression, specifically proportional odds and polytomous logistic regression.

6.4 How do I assess the impact of an individual variable on an outcome in a multivariable analysis?

In multivariable analysis, a regression coefficient for each variable is estimated by fitting the model to the data. The only difference between a multivariable regression coefficient and a bivariate regression coefficient (i.e., a coefficient from a regression model which contains only one independent variable) is that the coefficient and the intercept[114] are adjusted for all other variables that are in the model.

In the case of multiple logistic regression and proportional hazards analysis, the coefficients have a special meaning. The antilogarithm of the coefficient equals the odds ratio (for logistic regression) and the hazard ratio (for proportional hazards analysis). The hazard ratio (also known as the relative hazard) is a form of relative risk. More specifically, it is a rate ratio – a comparison of event rates in two groups.[115]

With interval independent variables the interpretation of the odds ratios/ hazard ratios derived from logistic regression or proportional hazards models can be confusing. As the odds ratio and hazard ratio represents the increase in

---

[112] See Scott, S.C., Goldberg, M.S., Mayo, N.E. Statistical assessment of ordinal outcomes in comparative studies. *J. Clin. Epidemiol.* 1997; 50: 45–55. Menard, S. *Applied Logistic Regression Analysis.* Thousand Oaks, CA: Sage Publications, 1995, pp. 80–90.

[113] See Feinstein, A.R. *Multivariable Analysis: An Introduction.* New Haven: Yale University Press, 1996, pp. 431–74.

[114] There is no intercept with proportional hazards regression.

[115] Spruance, S.L., Reid, J.E., Grace, M., Samore, M. Hazard ratio in clinical trials. *Antimicrob. Agents Chemother.* 2004; 48: 2787–92.

> With interval independent variables, the size of the odds ratio or hazard ratio is entirely dependent on how the interval variable is coded.

risk associated with a one-unit change in the interval independent variable, their size is entirely dependent on how the interval variable is coded.

For example, a study reported that the odds ratio for the effect of low-density lipoprotein (LDL) cholesterol on coronary artery calcification was 1.01 (95% CI = 1.00–1.02).[116] This may seem like a trivial effect until you notice that the odds ratio of 1.01 is for each increase of 1 mg/dl of LDL cholesterol. An increase of 40 mg/dl of cholesterol would produce an odds ratio of $(1.01)^{40}$ or 1.49. Although the change in the coding of the LDL cholesterol variable changes the odds ratio, it does not change the impact of LDL cholesterol on coronary artery calcification.

6.5 What assumptions underlie multivariable models?

Different assumptions underlie each of the three commonly used multivariable models.

The underlying assumption of linear regression is that as the independent variable increases (or decreases), the mean value of the outcome variable increases (or decreases) in a linear fashion. The only distinction between bivariate and multivariable linear regression is that with the latter you are assuming that the mean value of the outcome increases (or decreases) in a linear fashion with a linear *combination* of the independent variables. For example, a linear combination of age and body mass index is a good predictor of bone density among postmenopausal women.

Although multiple linear regression can only model a linear relationship between the independent variables and the outcome, it is possible to model non-linear relationships by transforming the variables so that the independent variables have a linear relationship to the outcome. Alternatively, non-linear relationships can be modeled using spline functions.[117]

Logistic regression models the probability of an outcome bounded by 0 and 1. The basic assumption is that each one-unit increase in a risk factor multiplies the odds of the outcome by a certain factor (the odds ratio of the risk factor), and that the effect of several risk factors is the multiplicative product of their individual effects. For example, if being male increases the risk of coronary artery disease by a factor of two (OR = 2.0) and having diabetes increases the risk of coronary artery disease by a factor of three (OR = 3.0) then men with

---

[116] O'Malley, P.G., Jones, D.L., Feuerstein, I.M., Taylor, A.J. Lack of correlation between psychological factors and subclinical coronary artery disease. *New. Engl. J. Med.* 2000; 343: 1298–1304.

[117] See: Harrell, F.E. *Regression Modeling Strategies: With Applications to Linear Models, Logistic Regression, and Survival Analysis.* New York: Springer-Verlag, 2001, pp. 18–24.

diabetes would be expected to be six times more likely to have coronary artery disease than women without diabetes.

Proportional hazards models assume that the ratio of the hazard functions for persons with and without a given risk factor is constant over the entire study period. This is known as the *proportionality assumption*.

Look back at Figures 5.7 and 5.9. Figure 5.7 fulfills the proportionality assumption because mortality steadily increases among persons who received transfusions compared to those who did not. In contrast, Figure 5.9 shows that event-free survival is initially lower among those persons who receive a stent, but in the latter part of the study (after about 150 days) event-free survival is higher among those who received stent. As the ratio between the hazard of an event with stenting and the hazard with angioplasty is not the same, the proportionality assumption is not fulfilled and you should not use proportional hazards models to analyse these data.[118]

---

[118] For more sophisticated methods of determining whether the proportionality assumption holds and methods of analyzing non-proportional data, see: Katz, M.H. *Multivariable Analysis: A Practical Guide for Clinicians* (2nd edition). New York: Cambridge University Press, 2005.

Sample size calculations

7.1 How do I determine the number of subjects needed for my study?

As explained in Section 2.11, sample size calculations should be done prior to performing your analysis. Nonetheless, I have placed this section after the sections on statistical analyses because you need to know what type of analysis you will be doing (e.g., chi-squared, *t*-test) to calculate the needed sample size.

For each type of statistical analysis you will need different elements (e.g., expected proportion, standard deviation) to determine the needed sample size.[119] These elements are explained in the sections below. Once you have these elements you can determine the needed sample size in one of the three ways:

1. use published tables;
2. use the formula;
3. use a software program.

Using published tables and formulas is adequate for calculating sample size for descriptive studies (univariate analysis). However, for more complicated designs it is better to use one of the available software packages.

Three software programs that are available free are:

1. Power and Sample Size (PS) by Dupont, W.D. and Plummer, W.D. (http://www.mc.vanderbilt.edu/prevmed/ps).
2. Statistical Considerations for Clinical Trials and Scientific Experiments by Schoenfeld, D. (http://hedwig.mgh.harvard.edu/sample_size/quan_measur/defs.html).
3. Simple Interactive Statistical Analysis (SISA) (http://home.clara.net/sisa/sampshlp.htm).

All the three software programs perform comparisons of unpaired means (*t*-test) and paired means (paired *t*-test). Of the three programs PS performs the widest

---

[119] For an easy to follow explanation of sample size, as well as tables and formulas for most of the univariate and bivariate analyses discussed here, see Hulley, S.B., Cummings, S.R., Browner, W.S., Grady, D., Hearst, N., Newman, T.B. *Designing Clinical Research* (2nd edition). Philadelphia, PA: Lippincott Williams & Wilkins, 2001, pp. 65–91. For a more detailed discussion on sample size see: Friedman, L.M., Furberg, C.D., DeMets, D.L. *Fundamentals of Clinical Trials* (3rd edition). New York: Springer, 1999, pp. 94–129.

array of calculations including sample size calculations for linear regression, survival analysis, and matched case control studies with an option of specifying more than one control per case. It requires downloading the software onto your computer; the other two are web based.

Unfortunately, none of these three packages perform sample size calculations for multivariable analysis. Sample size calculations for multiple linear regression and logistic regression can be performed using Power and Precision (http://www.power-analysis.com/specifications.htm). Although, it is not free, you can try it out for a free evaluation period.

As you will see in the sections below, sample size calculations require estimation of the result prior to performing the study. This may strike you as surprising and perhaps even troubling. After all, if you already knew the answer why would you perform the study? This is the paradox of sample size calculation. To perform a sample size calculation you have to estimate the very thing you are trying to learn.

There are three ways to resolve this paradox:
1. find comparable data;
2. conduct a pilot study;
3. base calculations on the smallest clinically meaningful difference.

Although there may be no published data with the exact population, conditions, and interventions as your planned study (if there is, choose a research question that has not already been answered!), you may be able to find data from a comparable population and/or set of circumstances.

If there are no comparable data, you will need to perform a pilot study. Pilot studies are useful for a variety of reasons. Besides providing an estimate of the effect size, pilot studies enable you to test recruitment, study procedures and instruments, and follow-up strategies. Many granting agencies will not fund your application unless you first demonstrate that your project is feasible.

The right size for a pilot study will depend on how novel your design and measures are (the more novel the larger the pilot). However, even pilot studies as small as 15–25 subjects can be invaluable in designing your full-scale project. And if you do not substantially change your study design or measures between the pilot and the full-scale study, you may be able to combine your pilot data with the data from the full-scale study to maximize sample size.

Basing sample size calculations on the smallest meaningful difference is a very practical strategy. After all, even if you could garner a large enough sample to demonstrate a smaller effect than one that would be clinically meaningful, what's the benefit of identifying a statistically significant but clinically trivial effect?

> The paradox of sample size calculation is that you have to estimate the very thing you are trying to learn.

> If possible, perform a pilot study to estimate effect size, test recruitment and follow-up strategies, and assess the quality of your measures.

Survey practicing physicians and/or patients to determine a clinically meaningful effect

For example, if you were performing a study where the outcome is blood pressure, a 20 mm decrease in blood pressure would certainly be clinically meaningful. A 10 mm decrease in blood pressure would also be clinically meaningful, but a 2 mm decrease would not be. Thus the smallest clinical effect that would be meaningful is something between 10 and 2 mm, perhaps a 5 mm reduction in blood pressure. To determine the minimal clinically important difference, survey practicing physicians and/or patients with the disease.[120]

When determining sample size requirements, remember you are calculating the number of subjects you will need for the analysis, not the number of subjects you will need to enroll. In almost all cases, you will need to enroll a larger number of subjects than that determined by your sample size calculation because you will have some subjects who will drop out of your study, be indeterminate on the outcome, have missing data on crucial covariates, etc.

Therefore, to determine how many persons you will need to enroll in your study, estimate the percentage of subjects you anticipate will have to be dropped from the analysis and increase your sample size accordingly. Here too pilot data on study retention will be very helpful.

To facilitate using the available software programs, I have organized the next sections in terms of the ingredients needed to perform a sample size calculation for each statistic.

Tip

Increase your calculated sample size to account for subjects who will be dropped from the analysis because of losses to follow-up, indeterminate outcome, or missing data.

7.2 How do I determine the sample size needed for univariate statistics?

Sample size determination for a univariate analysis is the easiest type of sample size calculation because you are not trying to test a hypothesis; you are simply determining the precision of each of your estimated values (e.g., a proportion, a mean). These estimated values are referred to as point estimates.

Intuitively, it should make sense to you that the larger the sample size, the greater the precision of the point estimate (because you are basing the estimate on extensive data). Conversely, the smaller the sample, the less precision (because you are basing the estimate on scanty data). Less precision means that there is a greater chance that the true value is far from the point estimate.

Although greater precision is always a good thing, identifying, enrolling, and evaluating subjects can be expensive and time consuming. You do not want to enroll more subjects than you need. For example, if you would be content to

---

[120] Man-Son-Hing, M., Laupacis, A., O'Rourke, K., et al. Determination of the clinical importance of study results. *J. Gen. Int. Med.* 2002; 17: 469–76.

Table 7.1. Required information for a sample size determination for univariate analyses

Dichotomous variable	Interval variable
Expected proportion	Expected standard deviation
Desired width of the confidence interval	Desired width of the confidence interval
Confidence level of interval	Confidence level of interval

estimate the prevalence of a disease in a population within 5–10% points of the true value you will need many fewer subjects than if you need to determine the prevalence within 1–2% points.

The information you will need to perform a power calculation for a univariate analysis with a dichotomous and an interval variable is shown in Table 7.1 and discussed in Sections 7.3 and 7.4.

7.3 How do I determine the sample size needed for a univariate analysis of a dichotomous variable (proportion)?

The three elements for determining the needed sample size for a univariate analysis of a dichotomous variable (Table 7.1) are:

1. *Expected proportion*

You will need more subjects to obtain the same precision for proportions near 50–50 (an even split) than for proportions at the extremes (e.g., 10–90%).

2. *Desired width of the confidence interval*

The desired width of the confidence interval is the range within which the true value would be expected to fall with repeated samples at a specified probability (e.g., 95% of the time; see #3). If, for example, you wanted your point estimate to have a precision of ±5%, the desired width of the confidence interval would be 10% (5% above and 5% below the point estimate equals a width of 10%).

3. *Confidence level of interval*

Choose the confidence level of the interval (e.g., 95%, 99%) based on how high a probability you want that the true value will fall within the confidence interval of the point estimate with repeated samples. Most commonly, 95% is selected. This would mean that with 95% of the repeated samples the true value is expected to fall within the confidence interval. If you want a higher probability that the true value will fall within the confidence interval with repeated samples, you can estimate your sample size needs assuming 99% confidence levels. This will require a larger sample size.

Tip

You will need more subjects to obtain the same precision for proportions near 50–50 (an even split) than for proportions at the extremes (e.g., 10–90%).

7.4 How do I determine the sample size needed for a univariate analysis of an interval variable (mean)?

The three elements for determining the needed sample size for a univariate analysis of an interval variable are (Table 7.1):

1. *Expected standard deviation*

For an interval variable you will need to estimate the expected standard deviation of the variable.

The more variability there is in a measurement (the greater the standard deviation), the greater the sample size you will need to have the same level of precision. The reason is that if your data points cover a wide range of values then a few points in either direction could strongly affect the point estimates.

> The more variability there is in a measurement, the larger the sample size needed to have the same level of precision.

For common variables (e.g., blood pressure) it should be relatively easy to find estimates of the standard deviation of the variable in the literature. When using published estimates remember that the standard deviation of a variable depends on the sample. If you have any doubt about whether this is true consider how much narrower the standard deviation of the variable of age would be if you measured it in an eighth grade class (all students would be around 13 years of age) versus if you measured it in a housing complex (residents would range from 0 to 90 years of age).

2. *Desired width of the confidence interval*

The principle for determining the width of the confidence interval for the mean is the same as with a proportion. The desired width of the confidence interval is the range within which the true value of the mean is expected to fall at a specified probability (see #3).

If, for example, you wanted the mean of blood pressure to have a precision of ± 5 mmHg, the desired width of the confidence interval would be 10 mmHg (5 mm above and 5 mm below the point estimate). With an interval variable, the desired confidence interval is in the units that the variable is measured (e.g., mm of Hg).

> **Tip**
> The standard deviation of a variable depends on the sample.

3. *Confidence level of interval*

The confidence level of the interval is usually set at 95%.

7.5 How do I determine the sample size needed for bivariate analysis?

As bivariate tests involve hypothesis testing, sample size calculation is more complicated with bivariate than univariate analysis.

The required elements for sample size determination for bivariate analyses are shown in Table 7.2.

Table 7.2. Required elements for sample size determination for bivariate analyses

Comparison of two proportions (association of two dichotomous variables) (chi-squared)	Comparison of two means (association of a dichotomous variable and a normally distributed interval variable) (*t*-test)	Association of two normally distributed interval variables (Pearson's correlation coefficient)	Comparison of two survival times (log-rank statistic)
Expected percentage in group 1	Effect size	Effect size	Effect size
Expected percentage in group 2	Standard deviation of interval variable		Accrual interval
Ratio of number of subjects in group 1 to number of subjects in group 2			Duration of trial
			Attrition rate
Alpha	Alpha	Alpha	Alpha
Power	Power	Power	Power

As was the case with univariate analyses, sample size calculations for bivariate analyses require that you estimate certain of the needed elements (expected percentages, effect size, standard deviation). As all four types of sample size calculation require that you specify the alpha and the power, I review these in this section and the other elements in Sections 7.6–7.9.

7.5.A Alpha

The alpha level is the probability of falsely rejecting the null hypothesis, that is rejecting the null hypothesis when it is actually true (Type I error).

As you are testing a hypothesis, you need to decide if your alternative hypothesis has one or two-tails. As discussed in Section 2.8, the only instance where it is appropriate to use a one-tailed test is when only one side of the alternative hypothesis is possible. This is rarely the case.

There is no correct alpha level. We choose an alpha level based on what is reasonable. Most studies accept a 5% chance of rejecting the null hypothesis when it is really true. Therefore, you will usually specify alpha as 0.05.

7.5.B Power

The power of a study is the probability of rejecting the null hypothesis if the actual effect is as large as the estimated effect size.

Although you might like a 100% chance of rejecting the null hypothesis when it is false (especially if you are going to commit 5 years of your life to the study!) research provides no such sure bets. We usually settle for a 0.80 or 0.90 probability (80% or 90% chance) of rejecting the null hypothesis if it is false.

Some tables and software programs for determining sample size ask for beta rather than power. Beta simply equals 1-power. It is the probability of failing to reject the null hypothesis when the difference between the groups really is as large or larger than the estimated effect size (Type II error).

7.6 How do I determine the sample size needed for comparison of two proportions (two dichotomous variables)?

The four needed elements[121] are:

1. *Expected percentages in group 1 and group 2*

It may surprise you that you have to specify the estimated proportion for both groups rather than simply the difference between the two groups (i.e., the effect size). The situation is analogous to sample size calculations for univariate analyses of dichotomous variables. You will remember (Section 7.3) that it takes a larger sample size to obtain the same precision for a proportion near to an even split (e.g., 50–50%) than for a proportion near to the extremes (e.g., 10–90%).

> It takes a larger sample size to demonstrate a statistically significant difference when the proportions are near 50% than when the proportions are at the extremes.

So too it takes a larger sample size to demonstrate that a 20% difference between two percentages is statistically significant when the percentages are near 50% (e.g., 40% versus 60%) than when the 20% difference occurs at the extremes (e.g., 10% versus 30%).

2. *Ratio of number of subjects in group 1 to the number of subjects in group 2*

The ratio of the number of subjects in one group to the number of subjects in the other group effects sample size. Specifically, the maximum efficiency (fewest total subjects needed to demonstrate a given effect) is achieved when you have equal numbers of subjects in each group. That being said, sometimes, it is markedly easier to obtain additional controls than cases. In such cases, adding additional controls, up to 4 per case, increases your power to demonstrate a given effect. (More than 4 controls per case results in very little incremental gain in power.)[122]

> Increasing controls beyond four per case results in very little incremental gain in power.

---

[121] Some statistical software packages will ask you to specify whether you want the continuity correction performed. Without the continuity correction, your sample size estimate will be for performance of a chi-squared test. With the continuity correction, your sample size estimate will be for performance of a Fisher's exact test. See Simple Interactive Statistical Analysis at http://home.clar.net/sisa/sampshlp.htm.

[122] Many software programs for sample size assume an equal number of cases and controls. For a simple method of approximating the decrease in the number of cases needed with increases in the number of controls, see Hulley, S.B., Cummings, S.R., Browner, W.S., Grady, D., Hearst, N., Newman, T.B. *Designing Clinical Research* (2nd edition). Philadelphia, PA: Lippincott Williams & Wilkins, 2001, pp. 78–9.

3. *Alpha*

see Section 7.5.A.

4. *Power*

see Section 7.5.B.

For example, Raine and colleagues evaluated the effect of direct access to emergency contraception on pregnancy rates.[123] Women were randomized into one of three groups: direct pharmacy access to emergency contraception (no prescription needed at pharmacy), direct provision of emergency contraception, or control (clinic access). The investigators formulated two null hypotheses: (1) there would be no difference in pregnancy rates between women with direct pharmacy access and controls; (2) there would be no difference in pregnancy rates between women with direct provision of emergency contraception and controls.

Based on prior research, the investigators assumed a 6-month pregnancy rate in the clinic access group and a 5% pregnancy rate in the pharmacy access and the direct provision group. They calculated that to have an alpha of 0.05 (assuming a two-sided test), and a power of 90%, they would need 620 women per treatment group. In the end, they enrolled 889 women in the pharmacy access group, 864 in the advance provision group, but only 344 in the clinic access group because during the time of the study, California law made it possible for all women to have pharmacy access without a prescription to emergency contraception. Although the study did not demonstrate a decrease in pregnancy among women randomized to pharmacy or direct access, the study was influential in showing no harm in making emergency contraception more freely available.

7.7 How do I determine the sample size needed for comparison of two means (association of a dichotomous variable with a normally distributed interval variable)?

The four needed elements[124] are:

1. *Effect size*

In the case of a comparison of two means, the effect size is the anticipated difference between the two means. It is expressed in the units of the interval variable.

2. *Standard deviation of the interval variable*

As with sample size determination for univariate analyses of interval variables (Section 7.4), you will need to estimate the expected standard deviation of your

---

[123] Raine, T.T., Harper, C.C., Rocca, C.H., et al. Direct access to emergency contraception through pharmacies and effect on unintended pregnancy and STIs. *J. Am. Med. Assoc.* 2005; 293: 54–62.

[124] Some statistical software programs ask you to specify whether you want the continuity correction performed for sample size calculations involving the comparison of means. Use the continuity correction when your sample size is small.

variable. The difference is that you will need to specify the standard deviation for each of the groups.

3. *Alpha*

see Section 7.5.A.

4. *Power*

see Section 7.5.B.

For example, recall the study of folate therapy on the risk of angiographic restensois after coronary-stent placement (Section 2.8). One of the end points of the study was luminal loss, defined as the difference between the minimal luminal diameter immediately after stenting and that at follow-up. The measurements were based on coronary angiography and were interval. In planning their study, the investigators calculated that to detect a luminal loss of 0.13 mm (effect size), assuming a standard deviation of 0.50 mm in each group, an alpha of 0.05 (assuming a two-sided test), and a power of 90%, they would need 622 patients (311 per group). To allow for dropouts they planned to enroll 650 patients, and ultimately enrolled 636 patients.

7.8 How do I determine the sample size needed for comparison of two normally distributed interval variables (Pearson's correlation coefficient)?

The three needed elements are:

1. *Effect size*

In the case of the correlation coefficient the effect size is the absolute value of the difference between the expected correlation and a correlation of zero. Therefore, if you expect the correlation to be -0.4 the effect size would 0.4. ($|-0.4 - 0| = 0.4$). We use the absolute difference because for a sample size calculation because it does not matter whether the correlation is positive or negative.

2. *Alpha*

see Section 7.5.A.

3. *Power*

see Section 7.5.B.

7.9 How do I determine the sample size needed for comparison of two survival times (log-rank statistic)?

The six needed elements are:

1. *Effect size*

Specify the median survival time for the two groups. The median survival time is the point at which 50% of the subjects have experienced the outcome (Section 4.6.A).

2. *Accrual interval*

For logistic reasons, most longitudinal studies enroll subjects over a period of time. (Depending on the number of subjects you need and the stringency of your enrollment criteria it may take years to enroll all your subjects.) Therefore, the starting dates for different subjects vary. As the ending date for all subjects is usually the same, the greater the delay in subject accrual (from the time the first subject is enrolled), the less observation time your study will have. With less observation time your study will have less power. Therefore, to calculate the sample size you will need to specify an accrual rate. The accrual rate can be constant (0.10 per month) or vary for each study interval (0.05 for the first month, 0.15 for the second month, etc.). The proportional accrual for each month should add up to 100% by the end of the study.

3. *Duration of trial*

Duration of the trial refers to the period of time from the date the first subject is enrolled to the end of the study. In general, the longer the duration of the study the greater the power because of increased observation time.

4. *Attrition rate*

Attrition rate refers to the frequency at which participants leave the study. To determine sample size, you will need to specify either a constant attrition rate (0.02 per month) or to vary the attrition rate for each study interval (0.01 for the first month, 0.03 for the second month, etc.). The greater the attrition rate, the lower the power of your study because you will have decreased observation time.

5. *Alpha*

see Section 7.5.A.

6. *Power*

see Section 7.5.B.

7.10 How do I determine the sample size needed for multivariable analyses?

Sample size calculation for multivariable analysis is complex and often requires consultation with a biostatistician. Nonetheless, there are a couple of rules of thumb that can help you get a sense of how large a sample size you will need.

First, determine the sample size needed to answer your question in a bivariate analysis (in other words, without adjustment for confounders) using one of the methods above. If you do not have enough subjects to answer your question in a bivariate analysis, you will not have enough subjects to answer your question in multivariable analysis.

Assuming you have enough subjects for a bivariate analysis, next see if you will have at least 10 outcomes (e.g., 10 subjects with a myocardial infarction or a diagnosis of cancer) per independent variable for multiple logistic regression and proportional hazards analysis. (In other words, if you have 50 outcomes, your study can accommodate 5 independent variables.) For multiple linear regression you need 20 subjects per independent variable. If not, your variable coefficients may have wide confidence intervals and your model may not be valid.[125]

Beyond this, to perform sample size calculations, use a software program that performs multivariable power calculations (e.g., Power and Precision available at www.power-analysis.com) and/or consult a biostatistician.

7.11 How do I determine the sample size needed to prove that two treatments are equal?

As discussed in Section 1.1, rejecting the null hypothesis (e.g., rejecting the hypothesis that there is no difference between two treatments) leads us to consider alternative hypotheses, such as that one treatment is superior to another.

But what if you are trying to prove equivalence? For example, what if you want to prove that two drugs are equally efficacious? This may be important if one drug is known to be less expensive, easier to administer, less likely to cause side effects or is preferable in some other way.

This type of trial is referred to an equivalence trial.[126] In planning an equivalence trial the goal is to power it such that you will have a high probability (ideally power of 0.90 or higher) of detecting a clinically meaningful difference if there is really one. If you do not find a difference, you can conclude that the two treatments are equivalent.

Sample size calculations for equivalence studies are generally done assuming a one-tailed test (because we are only interested in one side of the hypothesis – whether the new treatment is as good as the standard treatment).[127]

The major challenge of equivalence studies is that they require large sample sizes because you are trying to exclude small differences.

For example, the Columbus Investigators conducted an equivalence study comparing low-molecular-weight heparin to standard treatment for patients with

> **Tip**
>
> Equivalence studies require large sample sizes because you are trying to exclude small differences.

> To conduct an equivalence trial, set your power as high as possible (ideally, 0.90 or higher).

---

[125] Katz, M.H. *Multivariable Analysis: A Practical Guide for Clinicians* (2nd edition). New York: Cambridge University Press, 2005, pp. 77–81.

[126] Ware, J.H., Antman, E.M. Equivalence trials. *New Engl. J. Med.* 1997; 337: 1159–61.

[127] Some investigators prefer to use two-tailed tests with equivalence studies because it is more conservative. One-tailed equivalence studies may be referred to as "noninferiority" studies. For more on these two points see Parienti, J-J. "Tenofovir, equivalence, and noninferiority [letter]." *J. Am. Med. Assoc.* 2004; 292: 1951; Gallant, J.E., Staszewski, S., Pozniak, A.L., et al. "In Reply to tenofovir, equivalence, and noninferiority [letter]". *J. Am. Med. Assoc.* 2004; 292: 1951.

venous thromboembolism (blood clots).[128] Prior to their study, standard treatment for patients with thromboembolism was hospitalization for 5–10 days of intravenous unfractionated heparin with frequent blood draws to adjust the heparin dose. Low-molecular-weight heparin offers the advantage that it does not require hospitalization or blood monitoring. But is it equally effective?

The Columbus Group designed their study with the goal of having an 80% probability (power) of detecting a decrease (one-tailed test) in recurrence rate of 3% or greater with unfractionated heparin. In other words, if the trial showed a less than 3% difference in the rate of recurrence of thromboembolism the two treatments would be said to be equivalent.

The investigators found that the rate of recurrence was 4.9% with standard unfractionated heparin and 5.3% with low-molecular-weight heparin (0.4% difference indicates equivalence based on their predetermined criteria). The finding of equivalence has lead to the adoption of low-molecular-weight heparin as standard of care for venous thrombosis.

7.12 What if the sample size needed exceeds the sample size I can obtain?

If your sample size calculation indicates that you need more subjects than you can enroll, before abandoning your research question (which may ultimately be the best choice), consider the following options:

1. *Use a more sensitive marker of the outcome*
You may be able to identify an outcome that will be more sensitive to your intervention than the one you were originally planning to use. For example, death due to cardiovascular disease is a more sensitive marker of the efficacy of a cardiac treatment than death due to any cause. An episode of cardiac ischemia would be an even more sensitive marker of cardiac disease.

In general, interval variables are more sensitive than dichotomous variables and may enable you to answer your question with a smaller sample size. For example, systolic blood pressure in mg of Hg is a more sensitive measure of blood pressure than a dichotomous measure of hypertension (yes/no).

2. *Use repeated measurements*
Repeated measurements of the same subjects increases the number of observations without increasing the sample size (Section 5.10).

3. *Match cases and controls*
Matching decreases variability and thereby decreases the needed sample size. Also once you match for a variable, you will not need to statistically adjust for it in your analysis (Section 2.6.C). However, it is often hard to find matches.

---

[128] Columbus Investigators. "Low-molecular-weight heparin in the treatment of patients with venous thromboembolism". *New Engl. J. Med.* 1992; 337: 657–62.

4. *Use multiple controls*

You can decrease the number of cases needed by increasing the number of controls. However, the advantage of additional controls exists only up to four controls per case (Section 7.6).

5. *Relax your power*

For your sample size calculation, you may have set your power at 0.90 so that you would have a 90% probability of finding an association if there really is one. However, having learned that this will cause you to have to enroll an unmanageable number of subjects, you may be prepared to settle for an 80% chance of identifying an association if one exists.

6. *Perform your study in a population that is more likely to experience the outcome*

In studies of healthy persons few outcomes will occur. To increase the proportion of persons who experience the outcome (the maximal power occurs when half the persons experience the outcome) you could sample persons at higher risk for the disease. For example, rather than studying the impact of elevated cholesterol on the risk of myocardial infarction among healthy persons, you could study it among elderly men with hypertension and diabetes. Of course, then the results of your study will only be generalizable to elderly men with hypertension and diabetes.

7. *Increase the length of follow-up*

In a longitudinal study, the longer the follow-up time, the greater the power because there will be an increased number of outcomes. However, increasing the length of follow-up also has several drawbacks. The most serious is that longer studies lose more subjects to attrition. Although survival analysis can incorporate subjects who are lost to follow-up, the more subjects who are lost, the more you need to worry that the people who stay in the study are fundamentally different than those who are lost. In addition, longer studies are subject to temporal changes in treatment practices, are more costly, and delay learning the results.

8. *Use a proximal marker of outcome*

A proximal marker is highly predictive of a definitive outcome but occurs earlier and therefore results in more outcomes in a shorter follow-up period. For example, the definitive outcome for an HIV/AIDS drug treatment study is death. However, death is likely to occur in only a small number of subjects per year and a study using death as an outcome would require a very large sample size and/or a very long follow-up period. Instead, CD4 count can be used as a proximal marker of drug efficacy in HIV treatment studies. By setting a CD4 count threshold that constitutes "drug failure" (e.g., CD4 count <200 cells) studies can be performed more rapidly with smaller sample sizes.

Before using a proximal marker be sure that is accepted by the research community as highly predictive of the outcome. In the case of HIV/AIDS a large body of research indicates that there is a very strong association between decreasing CD4 count and increasing risk of death. It is because of this body of research that the United States Food and Drug Association accepts CD4 counts as evidence of drug efficacy for HIV/AIDS.

If none of these strategies work, find a new research question. Whatever you do, do not perform an underpowered study. Although there is a chance that you will uncover a larger effect than you estimated from your sample size calculation, what will you do if your study finds an effect similar or smaller in size than what you predicted? Publish it as a negative trial? But it is not a negative trial if it is underpowered! Publish it as an underpowered negative trial? But what good is that? Even if the two arms of the study produce identical results, with an underpowered study you may not be able to rule out a clinically significant difference. Avoid the problem by only undertaking adequately powered studies.

Tip

Do not undertake underpowered studies.

Studies of diagnostic and prognostic tests (predictive studies)

8.1 How do predictive studies differ from explanatory studies?

The major differences between predictive studies and explanatory studies are shown in Table 8.1.

> The goal of predictive studies is to predict the outcomes for *specific* patients while the goal of explanatory studies is to understand the *causes* of a particular outcome in a *population*.

The goal of predictive studies is to better diagnose illness and more accurately predict prognosis for *specific* patients. This is different from the goal of explanatory (etiologic) studies: to understand the *causes* of an illness or condition in a *population*.

As prediction models are used to make decisions for individual patients, they must predict outcomes with a high degree of certainty. For example, decision rules have been used to predict which patients presenting to an emergency department with possible cardiac ischemia will develop complications and therefore need intensive monitoring. One study found that an adaptation of the Goldman prediction rule correctly identified 89% of the patients who will develop complications.[129] If the clinical rule had only predicted half the patients with complications, it would never be used in clinical practice (and probably never would have been published, at least not in *Journal of American Medical Association*!). In contrast, all known risk factors for breast cancer account for only about 50% of breast cancer cases. Nonetheless, the results of these explanatory studies are still helpful to us in unraveling the causes of breast cancer.

> With predictive studies it does not matter whether the independent variable has a causal relationship with outcome.

When the goal is to predict outcome, it does not matter whether the independent variables have a causal relationship to the outcome. If a variable is closely associated with an outcome, such that its presence (or absence) predicts the outcome, that is sufficient. For example, ear lobe creases are a good predictor of coronary artery events (e.g., myocardial infarction, cardiac death) even

---

[129] Reilly, B.M., Evans, A.T., Schaider, J.J., et al. Impact of a clinical decision rule on hospital triage of patients with suspected acute cardiac ischemia in the emergency department. *J. Am. Med. Assoc.* 2002; 288: 342–50 (data reported are from the intervention group).

Table 8.1. Differences between predictive (diagnostic/prognostic) studies and explanatory studies

	Predictive studies	Explanatory studies
Goal	Predict outcome for individual patients	Reveal causes of disease in a population
Importance of model predicting outcome with high degree of certainty	High	Low
Nature of relationship between individual variables and outcome	Unimportant	Causal
Number of independent variables in the model	As few as possible to accurately predict outcome	As many as necessary to accurately assess the association of a risk factor with an outcome
Statistics used	Sensitivity, specificity, positive predictive value, likelihood ratio	Odds ratio, risk ratio
Theoretical basis	Bayes' theorem	Inferential statistics

though they do not cause coronary artery disease.[130] In contrast, with explanatory studies we strive to eliminate non-causal factors (e.g., confounding, bias) so that we can better understand the nature of the disease.

For predictive models to be incorporated into clinical practice, they need to be simple. Clinicians are unlikely to collect data on 15 different variables and plug the values into a calculator in order to decide what action to take. Also, the variables should be easily obtained. A predictive model that requires the result of a laboratory test not easily performed will not be widely used. For this reason, the predictive models that have gained the greatest popularity are those that use only a few easy to obtain variables.

> Predictive models should have as few variables as possible and the values of these variables should be easily obtained.

For example, the Ottawa rules are widely used in determining whether patients with ankle injuries need an X-ray because the rule requires determining only three things: (1) whether there is pain near the malleoli; (2) whether the patient could bear weight immediately and in the emergency department, and (3) whether there is bone tenderness at the posterior edge or tip of either malleolus.[131] This simple rule (if all three are negative no X-ray is necessary) has been shown to avoid about a third of X-rays without missing any fractures.

In contrast, with explanatory models we enter as many variables as necessary to accurately estimate the relationship between the predictors and the outcome. It is not unusual for an explanatory model to have 20 or 30 predictors. As long

---

[130] Elliott, W.J., Powell, L.H. Diagonal earlobe creases and prognosis in patients with suspected coronary artery disease. *Am. J. Med.* 1996; 100: 205–11.

[131] Stiell, I.G., Greenberg, G.H., McKnight, R.D., et al. Decision rules for the use of radiography in acute ankle injuries. *J. Am. Med. Assoc.* 1993; 269: 1127–32.

Table 8.2. Two-by-two table for calculating sensitivity and specificity

Test result	Disease present		Total
	Yes	No	
Positive	True positive	False positive	Subjects positive on the test
Negative	False negative	True negative	Subjects negative on the test
Total	Subjects with disease	Subjects without disease	All subjects

as the sample size is sufficient for the number of variables in the model (Section 7.10), and the right variables are included, there is no problem with having a larger model.

Predictive studies use different statistics than explanatory studies (Sections 8.2–8.6) and have a different theoretical basis (Section 8.6).

8.2 What are sensitivity and specificity?

Sensitivity and specificity are easiest to understand if you think of the data in terms of a two-by-two table as shown in Table 8.2.[132]

People who truly have the disease (e.g., coronary artery disease) will either be positive on the test (true positive) or negative (false negative). Sensitivity is the proportion of people with the disease who are positive on the test:

$$\text{sensitivity} = \frac{\text{subjects with true positive results}}{\text{total number of subjects with the disease}}$$

People who do not have the disease (no coronary artery disease) will either be positive on the test (false positive) or negative (true negative). Specificity is the proportion of subjects without the disease who are negative on the test:

$$\text{specificity} = \frac{\text{subjects with true negative results}}{\text{total number of subjects without the disease}}$$

Tip

Sensitivity is positive in disease and *specificity* is negative in health.

To distinguish sensitivity and specificity remember that sensitivity is positive in disease and specificity is negative in health.

---

[132] See: Fletcher, R.H., Fletcher, S.W., Wagner, E.H. *Clinical Epidemiology: The Essentials.* (3rd edition). pp. 48–60.

When it comes to diagnosing a patient, it is important to appreciate that no matter how sensitive a test is (even if it is 100%), it cannot help you to "rule in" a diagnosis. That is because sensitivity tells you nothing about the possibility that your positive test is a false positive. However, highly sensitive tests can be very helpful in "ruling out" a diagnosis because when a sensitive test is negative you know that the possibility that the result is a false negative is very small.

Conversely, no matter how specific a test is, it cannot help you to rule out a diagnosis. That is because specificity tells you nothing about the possibility that your negative result is a false negative. However, highly specific tests can be very helpful in "ruling in" a diagnosis because when a specific test is positive you know that the probability of the result being a false positive is low.

When you report sensitivity or specificity, show the 95% confidence intervals (CIs), as you would for any proportion (Section 4.3).

> **Tip**
>
> Sensitive tests (when negative) are helpful for "ruling out" disease and specific tests (when positive) are helpful for "ruling in" disease.

8.3 What are the positive and negative predictive values of a test?

> The positive predictive value is the probability that a person with a positive test result has the disease.

Neither sensitivity nor specificity tells you the likelihood that a positive test is a true positive. For this, you need to know the positive predictive value of the test. The positive predictive value is the probability that a person with a positive result actually has the disease. It is calculated from Table 8.2 as:

$$\text{positive predictive value} = \frac{\text{subjects with true positive results}}{\text{total number of subjects with positive results}}$$

Positive predictive value is especially relevant in evaluating the ability of a screening test to identify disease in healthy populations. Unlike tests performed in the setting of diagnosing disease, screening tests are performed on healthy populations. Commonly performed screening tests are occult blood testing of stool, mammograms, and prostate-specific enzyme.

In healthy populations the prior probability of disease is low. Consequently even tests with high sensitivity and specificity may produce as many (or more!) false positives as true positives.

The historical evolution in the use of HIV antibody tests illustrates this issue well. The anticipated results of compulsory premarital screening for HIV based on the characteristics of the HIV test in 1987 are shown in Table 8.3.[133]

The sensitivity of a positive result is 90% (1219/1348). The specificity is 99.9% (3,823,638/3,824,020). However the positive predictive value is only 76%

> **Tip**
>
> When the prior probability of disease is low, even tests with high sensitivity and specificity may produce as many or more false positives as true positives.

---

[133] Cleary, P.D., Barry, M.J., Mayer, K.H., et al. Compulsory premarital screening for the human immunodeficiency virus. *J. Am. Med. Assoc.* 1987; 258: 1757–62.

Table 8.3. Expected results of a premarital screening program for HIV in the USA based on the characteristics of the HIV test available in 1987

Test result	HIV infection		Total
	Yes	No	
Positive	1219 (true positive)	382 (false positive)	1,601
Negative	129 (false negative)	3,823,638 (true negative)	3,823,767
Total	1348	3,824,020	3,825,368

Data from Cleary, P.D., et al. Compulsory premarital screening for the human immunodeficiency virus. *J. Am. Med. Assoc.* 1987; 258: 1757–62.

(1219/1601). Twenty-four percent of the persons who would have been told that they were positive would actually have been uninfected! Based in part on this result, compulsory screening for persons marrying was not approved in the USA.

Ironically, since this analysis was performed the sensitivity of HIV antibody tests have improved such that HIV testing has a sensitivity of 99.9% and a specificity that approaches 100%. Given this, *voluntary* HIV testing in low-risk populations is appropriate.

The negative predictive value is the opposite of the positive predictive value. It is the probability that a person with a negative result does not have the disease. It is calculated from Table 8.2 as:

$$\text{negative predictive value} = \frac{\text{subjects with a true negative result}}{\text{all subjects with a negative result}}$$

The negative predictive value is an important metric when evaluating a test in populations with a high prevalence of disease.

To help distinguish positive and negative predictive values from sensitivity and specificity, remember that if your set up your two-by-two table to match Table 8.2, the positive and negative predictive values are calculated based on the rows while sensitivity and specificity are calculated based on the columns.

8.4 How do I determine the accuracy of a test?

The accuracy is the proportion of correct diagnoses. Looking back at Table 8.2 you will note that a "correct" diagnosis would be either a true positive or a true negative. Therefore, the accuracy of a test is:

$$\text{accuracy} = \frac{\text{true positive} + \text{true negative}}{\text{total sample size}}$$

A limitation of accuracy as a measure of the utility of a test is that it weighs the benefits of true positives and true negatives (or conversely the problems of false positives and false negatives) equally. But in many clinical situations, the implications of false positives and false negatives are not equal. In some cases, we are willing to have many false positives for the sake of never missing a diagnosis and in other cases we are willing to tolerate some false negatives so as not to falsely label people with a disease they don't have.

For example, the Goldman cardiac ischemia rule discussed in Section 8.1 correctly identified 89% of the patients who ultimately developed complications and therefore should have been admitted to a monitored bed.[134] However, 74% of the patients without cardiac complications were also referred to a cardiac bed. In other words, they set the threshold low so that they would send very few patients who would ultimately develop a complication to an unmonitored bed.

In contrast, with HIV testing the threshold of what is considered to be a positive test has been set high to avoid the possibility of incorrectly telling someone that they are HIV infected.

8.5 How do I calculate the characteristics of a test with an interval scale?

Calculating sensitivity, specificity, positive and negative predictive values requires having a dichotomous variable. What if you have an interval variable?

Determining the test characteristics of a continuous variable can be complicated because each potential cut-point will yield a different sensitivity, specificity, positive and negative predictive value.

For example, the prostate-specific antigen (PSA) test is used to screen for prostate cancer. It produces a continuous result reported in ng/ml. Hoffman and colleagues evaluated the accuracy of PSA testing by comparing the PSA of 930 men with biopsy proven prostate cancer to 1690 men who had a negative prostate biopsy.[135] The median PSA level for those with cancer (7.8 ng/ml) was significantly higher than for those without cancer (5.4 ng/ml) but there was considerable overlap between the groups, with the 25th and 75th percentiles being 4.9–14.2 ng/ml for the cancer group and 2.7–8.1 ng/ml for the men without cancer.

Table 8.4 shows the sensitivity, specificity, positive and negative predictive value of different cut-points of the PSA for prostate cancer.

Which cutoff of the PSA produces the best sensitivity, specificity, positive and negative predictive value? Trick question! There is no best cutoff because, as you

[134] Reilly, B.M., Evans, A.T., Schaider, J.J., et al. Impact of a clinical decision rule on hospital triage of patients with suspected acute cardiac ischemia in the emergency department. *J. Am. Med. Assoc.* 2002; 288: 342–50 (reported data are from the intervention group).

[135] Hoffman, R.M., Gilliland, F.D., Adams-Cameron, M., et al. Prostate-specific antigen testing accuracy in community practice. *BMC Fam. Prac.* 2002; 3: 19 (http://www.biomedcentral.com/1471-2296/3/19).

Table 8.4. Sensitivity, specificity, positive and negative predictive value of different cut-points of the PSA for prostate cancer

PSA cut-point (ng/ml)	Sensitivity (%)	Specificity (%)	Positive predictive value (%)	Negative predictive value (%)
1	98	9	37	91
2	95	20	39	88
3	91	26	40	84
4	86	33	41	81
5	75	44	42	76
6	63	57	45	74
7	56	66	48	73
8	49	74	51	72
9	42	80	53	71
10	38	84	56	71
15	23	93	67	69
20	17	97	78	68

Data from Hoffman, R.M., Gilliland, F.D., Adams-Cameron, M., et al. Prostate-specific antigen testing accuracy in community practice. *BMC Fam. Prac.* 2002; 3: 19 (http://www.biomedcentral.com/1471-2296/3/19).

can see from Table 8.4, you cannot maximize all the parameters. As the sensitivity increases the specificity decreases and as the positive predictive value increases the negative predictive value decreases. This will be the case with choosing the cutoff for any interval test result.

One way to resolve the dilemma of choosing a cut-point is to show the test characteristics at several different levels as in Table 8.4. In this way, a clinician can determine the characteristics of any particular test result. In other words, instead of deciding whether to pursue a biopsy based on knowing the positive predictive value associated with a result of the PSA value of ">4" (yes/no), the physician can make a recommendation based on the actual result.

The characteristics of a test at different cut-points can also be shown graphically using a receiver operating characteristic (ROC) curve.[136] An ROC curve for the test characteristics of the PSA test from the Hoffman study is shown in Figure 8.1.

The curve is constructed by plotting the sensitivity on the *y*-axis and (1 − specificity) on the *x*-axis. The further the curve is from the diagonal (dashed) line (the diagonal line represents a test that provides no information) and the closer it is to the upper left hand corner of the graph, the better the test it is.

---

[136] Hanley, J.A., McNeil, B.J. The meaning and use of the area under a receiver operating characteristic (ROC) curve. *Radiology* 1982; 143: 29–36. Hsiao, J.K., Bartko, J.J., Potter, W.Z. Diagnosing diagnoses: receiver operating characteristic methods and psychiatry. *Arch. Gen. Psychiat.* 1989; 46: 664–7.

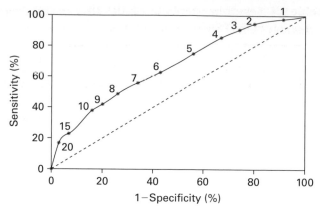

Figure 8.1   ROC curve for PSA testing. Reprinted from Hoffman, R.M., Gilliland, F.D.,
Adams-Cameron, M., et al. Prostate-specific antigen testing accuracy in
community practice. *BMC Fam. Prac.* 2002; 3: 19. (http://www.biomedcentral.
com/1471-2296/3/19)

Tests that are close to the upper left hand corner have high sensitivity and specificity (low values of 1 − specificity).

You can see from Figure 8.1 that the PSA is not a very good screening test. The
curve is not far from the diagonal line. This is consistent with the fact that the
25–75th quartile ranges for those with and without cancer are overlapping and
the fact that the test characteristics shown in Table 8.4 are not very high. In fact,
the US Preventive Services Task Force (USPSTF) concluded that there was
insufficient evidence to determine whether the benefits of screening with the
PSA outweighed the harms (e.g., unnecessary biopsies).[137]

In cases where you must choose a single cut-point for an interval test, it is best
to do it based on the clinical implications of false positive and false negative
results. When it is important not to miss a diagnosis, you need tests that are
highly sensitive. On the other hand, before subjecting patients to dangerous or
painful interventions, you need tests that are highly specific.

8.6 What is Bayes' theorem?

The point of predictive studies is to determine the probability of an event. This
is done using Bayes' theorem and likelihood ratios.

Bayes' theorem is a method of determining the probability of an event based
on the: (1) pretest probability of the event and (2) the information added by a

---

[137] USPSTF. Screening for prostate cancer: recommendation and rationale. *Ann. Int. Med.* 2002; 137: 915–16.

Definition

Bayes' theorem is a method for determining the probability of an event based on the pretest probability of the event and the information added by a test.

test.[138] It is the theoretical basis for predictive models (in contrast to explanatory models which are based on inferential statistics).

Although Bayes' theorem sounds complicated, we incorporate Bayes' theorem in our everyday clinical decision-making. For example, imagine that two patients roll into the emergency department: Ms. Jones and Mr. Smith. They have identical complaints of substernal chest pain. Ms. Jones is a 34-year-old woman, non-smoker, with no prior medical history. Mr. Smith is a 55-year-old man with hypertension, diabetes, elevated cholesterol, and a 25-pack year history of smoking. As the patients have acute chest pain, the nurse immediately obtains an electrocardiogram (EKG) on both. As she hands them to you she rattles off a one-sentence description of the patients.

Now, before you even look at the EKGs, you have a different sense of these two patients. Although it is not impossible that Ms. Jones is having a myocardial infarction, the likelihood that a pre-menopausal non-smoking woman has heart disease is very low. In Bayesian terms, she has a low *pretest probability* of coronary artery disease. The pretest probability is the likelihood of a condition (e.g., myocardial infarction) prior to considering the new evidence (e.g., EKG).

The pretest probability is the likelihood of the condition prior to considering new evidence.

In contrast, Mr. Smith has a high pretest probability of having a myocardial infarction because he has four risk factors (male, hypertension, diabetes, elevated cholesterol). To know the true pretest probability for both Ms. Jones and Mr. Smith, you would have to conduct a study looking at the proportion of patients presenting to an emergency department with risk factor profiles similar to theirs who turn out to have a myocardial infarction. However, even without knowing the exact pretest probability, we can say with certainty that it is much higher for Mr. Smith than Ms. Jones.

A diagnostic test, in this case the EKG, gives you a new probability of outcome, the posttest probability, which is conditional on the pretest probability and the new information, as shown in Figure 8.2.

The posttest probability is the likelihood of a condition given the pretest probability of the condition and the information added by the test.

For example, the low pretest probability for myocardial infarction for Ms. Jones would become higher if she had 4 mm of ST elevation in leads V1–V4. The high pretest probability for Mr. Smith would become lower if he had a normal EKG.

How different the posttest probability is from the pretest probability depends on the likelihood ratio of the test. The likelihood ratio for a dichotomous test is

---

[138] Although I refer to the new information as a test, it can be a series of tests, a piece of information derived from interviewing the patient (e.g., Did the chest pain start when you were exerting yourself?), or a physical finding on examination (e.g., a third heart sound). See Fletcher, R.H., Fletcher, S.W., Wagner, E.H. *Clinical Epidemiology: The Essentials* (3rd edition). Philadelphia: Lippincott Williams & Wilkins, 1996, p. 43.

pretest probability + information from test ⟶ posttest probability

Figure 8.2
Use of Bayes' theorem to determine the likelihood of outcome from the pretest probability and the result of the test.

expressed in terms of a positive test result (the likelihood ratio of a positive test) or a negative test result (the likelihood ratio of a negative test).

The likelihood ratio[139] of a positive test equals:

$$\text{likelihood ratio of a positive test } = \frac{\text{probability of a positive test result in someone with the disease}}{\text{probability of a positive test in someone without the disease}}$$

Note that the numerator "probability of a positive test result in someone with the disease" is the sensitivity of the test (Section 8.2). The denominator is a little less obvious. If the probability of a negative test result in someone without the disease is specificity, than the "probability of a positive test result in someone without the disease" is: $1 -$ specificity.

$$\text{likelihood ratio of a positive test } = \frac{\text{sensitivity}}{(1 - \text{specificity})}$$

A likelihood ratio of a positive test >1 signifies an increased probability that a patient with a positive result has the disease. A likelihood ratio of a positive test of <1 signifies a decreased probability that the patient has the disease.

The likelihood ratio of a negative test equals:

$$\text{likelihood ratio of a negative test } = \frac{(1 - \text{sensitivity})}{\text{specificity}}$$

A likelihood ratio of a negative test >1 signifies an increased probability that a patient with a negative result has the disease. A likelihood ratio of a negative test of <1 signifies a decreased probability that the patient has the disease with a negative result on the test.

When tests are measured on an interval scale likelihood ratios are expressed in terms of a particular cutoff of that test (e.g., positive likelihood ratio of a

---

[139] The term likelihood ratio has a different meaning when used in the context of logistic regression or proportional hazards regression. In that context, it is the ratio of the likelihood that the data represent the null hypothesis to the likelihood the data represent the alternative hypothesis.

cholesterol of 240 mg/dL or more). As with sensitivity and specificity, you can determine a positive likelihood ratio for each different cutoff of an interval variable.

To use likelihood ratios to determine the posterior probability of a disease you must first convert the pretest probability to the pretest odds. This is not difficult to do:

$$\text{pretest odds} = \frac{\text{pretest probability}}{(1 - \text{pretest probability})}$$

Once you have the pretest odds you multiply it by the likelihood ratio to determine the posttest odds.

$$\text{pretest odds} \times \text{likelihood ratio} = \text{posttest odds}$$

You can then convert the odds back into a probability:

$$\text{posttest probability} = \frac{\text{posttest odds}}{(1 + \text{posttest odds})}$$

For example, let us say that a 4-year-old child comes into your office with an earache. The prevalence of acute otitis media in a child this age seen in an outpatient setting has been estimated to be 20%.[140] You examine the child's ear. The color of the eardrum is cloudy. How likely is it that the child has otitis media?

First, convert the prior prevalence to prior odds:

$$\text{prior odds} = \frac{0.20}{(1 - 0.20)} = \frac{0.20}{0.80} = 0.25$$

Note that the likelihood ratio for a cloudy eardrum is 34 (Table 8.5).[141] You therefore multiply the prior odds by the likelihood ratio to obtain the posterior odds.

$$\text{posttest odds} = 0.25 \times 34 = 8.5$$

Finally, convert the posttest odds to posttest probability:

$$\text{posttest probability} = \frac{8.5}{9.5} = 0.89$$

[140] Rothman, R., Owens, T., Simel, D.L. Does this child have acute otitis media? *J. Am. Med. Assoc.* 2003; 290: 1633–40.

[141] From Rothman, R., Owens, T., Simel, D.L. Does this child have acute otitis media? *J. Am. Med. Assoc.* 2003; 290: 1633–40 based on data originally reported by Karma, P.H., Penttila, M.A., Sipila, M.M., et al. Otoscopic diagnosis of middle ear effusion in acute and non-acute otitis media: I. the value of different otoscopic findings. *Int. J. Pediatr. Otorhinolaryngol.* 1989; 17: 37–49.

Table 8.5. Likelihood ratios for three major signs of otitis media

Signs of otitis media	Likelihood ratio (95% CI)
Color	
Cloudy	34 (28–42)
Distinctly red	8.4 (6.7–11)
Slightly red	1.4 (1.1–1.8)
Normal	0.2 (0.19–0.21)
Position	
Bulging	51 (36–73)
Retracted	3.5 (2.9–4.2)
Normal	0.5 (0.49–0.51)
Mobility	
Distinctly impaired	31 (26–37)
Slightly impaired	4.0 (3.4–4.7)
Normal	0.2 (0.19–0.21)

From Rothman, R., Owens, T., Simel, D.L. Does this child have acute otitis media? *J. Am. Med. Assoc.* 2003; 290: 1633–40 based on data originally reported by Karma, P.H., Penttila, M.A., Sipila, M.M., et al. Otoscopic diagnosis of middle ear effusion in acute and non-acute otitis media: I. The value of different otoscopic findings. *Int. J. Pediatr. Otorhinolaryngol.* 1989; 17: 37–49.

Seeing that the child's eardrum is cloudy changes the probability that the ear is infected from 0.20 to 0.89 and would likely result in prescribing antibiotics for the child.

An important feature of likelihood ratios is that they can be used to calculate the posterior probability of a disease based on the results of multiple diagnostic tests by multiplying the likelihood ratios together:

> To use multiple likelihood ratios to determine the posttest odds of an outcome, the likelihood ratios must be based on test results that are independent of one another.

$$\text{pretest odds} \times \frac{\text{likelihood}}{\text{ratio test 1}} \times \frac{\text{likelihood}}{\text{ratio test 2}} \times \frac{\text{likelihood}}{\text{ratio test 3}} = \text{posttest odds}$$

This is potentially useful because in most clinical situations we have more than one relevant test result and wish to use each piece of information to determine a patient's diagnosis or prognosis. However, to incorporate more than one likelihood ratio in this way the likelihood ratios have to be based on test results that are independent of one another.

Unfortunately, many test results have not been demonstrated to be independent of one another. For example, it is not known whether the test results underlying the likelihood ratios shown in Table 8.5 are independent of one another. Therefore, you cannot simply multiply them by one another.

8.7 How do I choose the best standard for predictive studies?

When you are performing a predictive study, you need to define what standard you will use for deciding that a subject has a particular disease or outcome. The standard should be chosen prior to the start of the study to avoid biasing your choice by using information you have learned in the data collection process.

Ideally, you should test the characteristics of a diagnostic or prognostic test against the most rigorous standard available. This is referred to as the gold standard.

However, the most rigorous standard may not be feasible because of safety concerns, acceptability to subjects, and cost. Indeed, different investigators in the same field may choose different standards based on their sense of what is feasible.

For example, two studies of the ability of helical computed tomography (CT) to diagnose pulmonary embolisms (clots in the lung) used different standards. Qanadli and colleagues used the gold standard: pulmonary arteriography.[142] In contrast van Strijen and colleagues used a clinical standard.[143] Instead of subjecting patients to angiography, an invasive test that can result in serious adverse reactions, they performed compression ultrasonography to check for blood clots in the legs of subjects who had normal helical CT scans (identifying a blood clot in the leg makes a pulmonary embolism more likely and is a reason for initiating anticoagulation regardless of whether the patient has a pulmonary embolism). In addition, they followed subjects clinically for development of respiratory symptoms consistent with pulmonary embolism.

If you intend to use the clinical course of your patients rather than the gold standard to determine the clinical outcome it is critical that you:

1. Set the criteria of what will determine an outcome a priori (prior to the start of the study).
2. Create an independent committee to review the clinical course of the subjects.
3. Maintain close contact with your subjects.

In the case of the study by van Strijen and colleagues, there was an independent committee that reviewed all clinical data and no subjects were lost to follow-up.

---

[142] Qanadli, S.D., Hajjam, M.E., Mesurolle, B., et al. Pulmonary embolism detection: prospective evaluation of dual-section helical CT versus selective pulmonary arteriography in 157 patients. *Radiology* 2000; 217: 447–55.

[143] Van Strijen, M.J.L., de Monye, W., Schiereck, J., et al. Single-detector helical computed tomography as the primary diagnostic test in suspected pulmonary embolism: a multicenter clinical management study of 510 patients. *Ann. Intern. Med.* 2003; 138: 307–14.

8.8 What population should I use for determining the predictive ability of a test?

Predictive models should be tested in samples that are similar to the ones that the model will be used in. In particular, the prevalence and severity of disease, along with the prevalence and severity of diseases that mimic the disease under study, will all affect the performance of the model.

If you choose a sample where persons are likely to have advanced disease, the sensitivity of a test will likely be higher than it will in samples where the disease is at an earlier stage. Conversely, if you select a sample of very healthy controls, the specificity of the model will be higher than in populations where there is a high prevalence of other diseases that could mimic the disease you are studying. This is referred to as spectrum bias. Spectrum bias occurs when predictive models are tested on samples that are not representative of the person for whom the model will be used.[144]

> **Tip**
>
> To avoid spectrum bias test your predictive model in a setting similar to the one in which the model will be used.

8.9 How is validity determined for predictive studies?

Even if your predictive model has high sensitivity, specificity, and accuracy, was developed using the accepted gold standard, and was tested in the relevant population, it is unlikely to be adopted in clinical practice until it has been validated on a second sample. The reason is that models derived from one sample usually do not perform as well with new data. Therefore it is best to test the validity of the model by collecting a second set of data and see how well the model developed on the first dataset predicts outcome in the second dataset. When this is impossible, you can simulate a second wave of data collection by using one of three available methods for validating a model with a single dataset: split-group, jackknife, or bootstrap technique.[145]

---

[144] For more on the sources of variation and bias that affect diagnostic tests see: Whiting, P., Rutjes, A.W.S., Reitsma, J.B., et al. Sources of variation and bias in studies of diagnostic accuracy. *Ann. Intern. Med.* 2004; 140: 189–202; Fletcher, R.H., Fletcher, S.W., Wagner, E.H. *Clinical Epidemiology: The Essentials* (3rd edition). pp. 54–5; Hulley, S.B., Cummings, S.R., Browner, W.S., Grady, D., Hearst, N., Newman, T.B. *Designing Clinical Research* (2nd edition). Philadelphia: Lippincott Williams & Wilkins. 2001, pp. 179–80.

[145] For more on validating diagnostic and prognostic models see Katz, M.H. *Multivariable Analysis: A Practical Guide for Clinicians* (2nd edition). Cambridge: Cambridge University Press, 2005, pp. 179–83.

Statistics and causality

9.1 When can statistical association establish causality?

Never! Not even when you have performed the most elegant study possible and have obtained statistically significant results! Establishing causality is difficult because even after eliminating chance as the explanation of an association, you still have to eliminate confounding, bias, effect–cause, and bias.

Although association does not equal causality, there are a number of methods that can be implemented both prior to and after data collection that increase the chance that an association is causal (Table 9.1). These strategies are particularly important for non-randomized studies because of the many sources of potential confounding and bias inherent in this design.

9.1.A Prior research

Associations that have been documented in prior studies are more likely to be true than completely novel associations. In Bayesian terms, when prior studies have shown an association to be present, there is a higher prestudy (pretest) probability that the finding is true.

> With novel associations, be especially rigorous in assessing the possibility that the association is spurious.

Of course, someone has to be the first to document a true association, and science would not progress much if we all ignored new associations. But if you are the first to uncover an association, rigorously ask yourself the questions that are listed in Table 9.1 and report the results cautiously.

For example, Habu and colleagues conducted a study to assess whether administration of vitamin K_2 would prevent bone loss in women with viral cirrhosis of the liver. After the study was completed, 40 of the 43 original participants agreed to participate in a longer trial. The investigators found that women who had been randomized to vitamin K_2 in the original study were significantly less likely to develop hepatocellular carcinoma (OR = 0.13; 95% confidence

Table 9.1. Tests for assessing the likelihood that a statistical association is causal[146]

Criteria	Methods for assessing or strengthening causal inference
Is it consistent with prior research?	Literature search
Is it biologically plausible?	Understanding the pathophysiology
Is there a dose–response relationship?	Trend test
Is the effect strong?	Magnitude of risk ratio, rate ratio, odds ratio, hazard ratio
Have you excluded:	
Confounding?	Randomization, matching, stratification, multivariable analysis
Effect–cause?	Longitudinal design, long interval between ascertainment of risk factor and disease, rigorous screening for outcome at baseline examination
Bias?	Randomization, blinding

interval $= 0.02$–0.99; $P = 0.05$).[147] Since the result was unexpected, the study was small and performed in a single center, and three of the cases of hepatocellular carcinoma in the control group were diagnosed within a year of enrolment (the subjects may have had occult disease at the time of enrollment), the authors were appropriately cautious in reporting their results. Rather than recommend that women with viral cirrhosis take vitamin K_2 they concluded that their results "must be confirmed by multicenter randomized controlled studies with the prevention of hepatocellular carcinoma by vitamin K_2 as the primary end point."

9.1.B Biologic plausibility

Biologically plausibility also increases the probability that an association is causal. For example, the fact vitamin K_2 is known to play a role in controlling cell growth and has been shown to inhibit growth of human cancer cell lines, strengthens the possibility that the association between vitamin K_2 and decreased cases of hepatocellular cancer identified by Habu and colleagues is causal.

On the other hand, lack of a biological explanation may simply reflect our collective ignorance. For example, many medicinal plants were known to be

---

[146] These strategies are derived from the criteria for assessing causal inference articulated by Hill, A.G. The environment and disease: association or causation? *Proc. Roy. Soc. Med.* 1965; 58: 295–300.

[147] Habu, D., Shiomi, S., Tamori, A., et al. Role of vitamin K_2 in the development of hepatocellular carcinoma in women with viral cirrhosis of the liver. *J. Am. Med. Assoc.* 2004; 292: 358–61.

Table 9.2. Dose–response relationship between respiratory symptoms and workplace smoked exposure

Hours*	Odds ratio (95% Confidence Intervals)				
	≤4	>4–16	>16–48	>48	P for trend
Men	1.7 (1.4–2.1)	2.3 (1.8–2.8)	2.7 (2.2–3.4)	3.2 (2.5–4.0)	<0.001
Women	1.0 (0.6–1.7)	1.6 (0.9–2.8)	2.7 (1.5–4.9)	2.0 (1.1–3.4)	<0.001

* Hours based on number of cigarettes smoked nearby multiplied by the number of hours exposed per day at work. The odds ratios in this table are adjusted for a number of possible confounders using multiple logistic regression. Data are from: Lam, T.H., et al. "Environmental tobacco smoke exposure among police officers in Hong Kong." *J. Am. Med. Assoc.* 2000; 284: 756–63.

effective (e.g., foxglove, curare) long before the mechanism of action was determined. Also, hypothesized mechanisms of action may be wrong.

9.1.C Dose–Response

Identifying a dose–response relationship strengthens causal inference. For example, Lam and colleagues studied the impact of workplace smoke exposure on the respiratory status of non-smoking police officers.[148] Table 9.2 shows the odds ratio for any respiratory symptom based on the number of hours of workplace smoke exposure.

Note that as exposure increases the odds of having respiratory symptoms increases for both men and women. The increase is statistically significant based on the *P* for trend. The *P* for trend tests the hypothesis that there is no linear relationship between the workplace exposure and the risk of respiratory symptoms. Since the *P*-value is small we can reject the null hypothesis and assume that there is a linear relationship between workplace smoke exposure and respiratory symptoms. The finding of a dose–response relationship increases the likelihood that workplace smoke exposure is causally related to the respiratory symptoms.[149]

9.1.D Strength of effect

Stronger effects are more likely to be causal, in part, because confounders operate indirectly (see Figure 6.1) and are therefore less likely to produce strong effects. Some authors suggest that a relative risk (e.g., risk ratio, rate ratio, relative

---

[148] Lam, T.H., Ho, L.M., Hedley, A.J. Environmental tobacco smoke exposure among police officers in Hong Kong. *J. Am. Med. Assoc.* 2000; 284: 756–63.

[149] Astute readers will note that among women the linear trend is not perfect: the >48 cigarette-hours had a lower odds ratio than the >16–48 h. However, the overall trend is upward. For more on tests for linear trend see: Vittinghoff, E., Glidden, D.V., Shiboski, S.C., McCulloch, C.E. *Regression Methods in Biostatistics.* New York: Springer, 2005, pp. 82–3.

hazard) of 3.0–4.0 or higher (or a relative risk of <0.33 for protective effects) makes it unlikely that confounding is the exclusive explanation of the increased risk.[150] Although any cut-off is arbitrary, the principle is correct.

For example, one of the reasons we feel so certain that cigarette smoking causes lung cancer even though there are no randomized studies on this issue is that the relative risk of lung cancer with smoking is very high. This was demonstrated by Thun and colleagues. Using a prospective cohort design and a proportional hazards analysis to adjust for confounders, they found that the relative hazard of smoking for cancer of the trachea, bronchus, lung was 21.3 (95% CI 17.7–25.6) among current male smokers and 12.5 (95% CI 10.9–14.3) among current women smokers.[151]

Although stronger effects are more likely to be true, if the true relative risk between a risk factor and an outcome is 2.0, then no study will ever meet this criterion. Therefore, you should not assume that any association with a relative risk of <3.0 is due solely to confounding.

9.1.E Exclude confounding

In assessing whether your association could be due to confounding, consider both unknown (or unmeasured) and known confounders. Remember that only randomization can eliminate confounding due to unknown confounders (Section 2.4).

Even for known confounders, statistical adjustment using multivariable analysis is an imperfect method of eliminating confounding. This point is often missed by investigators who mistakenly believe that because they have included a potential confounder in their multivariable model, they have eliminated confounding due to that variable. But statistical adjustment for known confounders is never perfect. Your measure of the confounder may not perfectly capture the underlying confounder. Your model may not perfectly fit your data (no model does!). Therefore, even though you have "adjusted" for a confounder by including it in your model, you may still have residual confounding.

> **Tip**
>
> Even after statistical adjustment, you can still have residual confounding.

9.1.F Exclude reverse causality (effect–cause)

Reverse causality (effect–cause) is primarily a problem with cross-sectional designs because the risk factor and the outcome are measured at the same time (Section 2.6.A). For example, several cross-sectional studies have shown an

---

[150] Taubes, G. Epidemiology faces its limits. *Science* 1995; 269: 164–9.
[151] Thun, M.J., Apicella, L.F., Henley, S.J. Smoking vs other risk factors as the cause of smoking-attributable deaths. *J. Am. Med. Assoc.* 2000; 284: 706–12.

association between having a case manager and receiving supportive services among HIV-infected persons. Advocates have used these studies as justification for funding case management programs, pointing out that having a case manager results in patients receiving needed services. However, these studies were vulnerable to the criticism of reverse causality, specifically the possibility that receiving services led to getting a case manager (because many service organizations automatically assign case managers to patients who request services).

To resolve this issue colleagues and I used a longitudinal probability sample of HIV-infected persons (HIV Cost and Services Utilization Study, HCSUS).[152] We identified two groups: (1) subjects with unmet needs and case managers at baseline and (2) subjects with unmet needs and no case managers at baseline. We found that contact with a case manager at baseline was associated with a higher likelihood that unmet needs were fulfilled by the time of the follow-up visit. By requiring that the case manager be in place prior to the unmet need being fulfilled, we excluded the possibility that receiving services resulted in getting a case manager and thereby strengthened the argument that there was a causal relationship between having a case manager and receiving needed services.

Even with longitudinal studies, reverse causality may be operating if the disease you are studying has a subclinical form. This is why it is important to intensively screen for subclinical disease at the start of a study. For example, in Section 2.3.A I discussed the evidence supporting a relationship between participating in challenging cognitive activities and not developing dementia. But what if effect–cause is operating? Could it be that persons with undiagnosed dementia are less likely to engage in challenging cognitive activities? When such people are observed years later the dementia has progressed and the lack of engagement in challenging cognitive activities is assumed to be one of the reasons. To guard against this possibility, the investigators tested all subjects at baseline for dementia using a standardized instrument that closely correlates with the stages of Alzheimer's disease.

9.1.G Exclude bias

Of potential threats to causality, bias can be the most difficult to assess because there are so many sources of potential bias. Remember from Section 1.1 that bias is systematic error in the design or execution of a study.[153] Selection bias may

---

[152] Katz, M.H., Cunningham, W.E., Fleishman, J.A., et al. Effect of case management on unmet needs and utilization of medical care and medications among HIV-infected persons. *Ann. Int. Med.* 2001; 135: 557–65.

[153] For more on bias, see Szklo, M., Nieto, F.J. *Epidemiology: Beyond the Basics.* Gaithersburg, Maryland: Aspen Publication, pp. 125–76; Hulley, S.B., Cummings, S.R., Browner, W.S., Grady, D., Hearst, N., Newman, T.B. *Designing Clinical Research* (2nd edition). Philadelphia: Lippincott Williams & Wilkins, 2001, pp. 126–8.

occur in sampling of subjects or assignment to study groups (e.g., sicker persons being steered to a particular treatment group); bias may occur due to subjects with a disease being more likely to remember exposures (recall bias) or due to subjects answering questions the way they think the investigators want them to (i.e., social desirability bias); bias may occur due to interviewers probing more deeply with subjects they think likely to have had an exposure; observer bias occurs when the investigator draws a conclusion about a participant based on collateral information about the patient (e.g., investigator assumes that an AIDS patient is taking zidovudine because the patient has an elevated MCV level).

The best way to minimize bias is through careful study design. However, even if you perform a randomized placebo-controlled trial there are still potential sources of bias (e.g., subjects submitting their pills to a private laboratory to unblind their assignment). As a researcher, all you can do is minimize the sources of bias, test the impact of bias in your study (e.g., if study dropout is high among older persons, test your results in younger persons; if the association holds then you know it cannot be due solely to bias due to dropout among older persons); and honestly report the biases of your study.

9.1.H Strengthening causal associations: putting it all together and getting it wrong!

The association between estrogen use and Alzheimer's disease provides a perfect example of how to strengthen causal associations and get it wrong!

Five observational studies showed that estrogen use was associated with decreased development of Alzheimer's disease (**prior research**).[154] Estrogen is known to have positive effects on the brain including reducing beta-amyloid accumulation, enhancing neurotransmitter release and action, and protecting against oxidative damage (**biologic plausibility**).[155] The prospective longitudinal study performed by Tang and colleagues carefully evaluated subjects on enrollment to exclude incipient Alzheimer's disease (**exclude reverse causality**). All five of the studies used multivariable analysis to control for possible confounders such as age, education, ethnicity, age at menarche, age at menopause, and apolipoprotein E genome (**exclude confounding**). To test for bias due to

---

[154] Tang, M.-X., Jacobs, D., Stern, Y., et al. Effect of oestrogen during menopause on risk and age at onset of Alzheimer's disease. *Lancet* 1996; 348: 429–32; Baldereschi, M., De Carlo, A., Lepore, V., et al. Estrogen-replacement therapy and Alzheimer's disease in the Italian longitudinal study on aging. *Neurology* 1998; 50: 996–1002; Zandi, P.P., Carlson, M.C., Plassman, B.L., et al. Hormone replacement therapy and incidence of Alzheimer disease in older women. *J. Am. Med. Assoc.* 2002; 288: 2123–9; Paganini-Hill, A., Henderson, V.W. Estrogen deficiency and risk of Alzheimer's disease in women. *Am. J. Epidemiol.* 1994; 140: 256–61; Kawas, C., Resnick, S., Morrison, A., et al. A prospective study of estrogen replacement therapy and the risk of developing Alzheimer's disease: The Baltimore Longitudinal Study of Aging. *Neurology* 1997; 48: 1517–21.

[155] Yaffe, K. Hormone therapy and the Brain: Déjà vu all over again? *J. Am. Med. Assoc.* 2003; 289: 2717–18.

excluding women with Parkinson's disease or stroke, Tang and colleagues compared hormone use among excluded women to that of women included in the study and found no differences (**exclude bias**). The protective effect was strong (OR < 0.33) in the study by Baldereschi and colleagues (**strength of effect**). Three studies (Tang and colleagues, Paganini-Hill and Henderson, and Zandi and colleagues) found an association between longer duration of estrogen use and decreased incidence of Alzheimer's disease (**dose–response relationship**).

However, when a randomized clinical trial was completed, it showed that estrogen plus progestin therapy actually increased the risk of dementia.[156] How could the observational studies been so wrong? The reason for the discrepancy between the observational data and the randomized controlled trial is unknown. The most likely explanation is confounding due to an unmeasured factor such as healthful life-style behavior.

9.2 Can the results be statistically significant and clinically unimportant?

Absolutely! The reason is that statistical significance is heavily affected by sample size. If you have any doubt remember the coin toss example (Section 1.1). Having 60% of the tosses land on heads is sufficient evidence to conclude the coin is equally weighted if you have 100 tosses but not if you only have 10 tosses.

Why is sample size such an important determinant of statistical significance? The reason is that you are more likely to correctly characterize a population if you assess a large number of its members than if you assess a small number of members.

> You are more likely to correctly characterize a population if you assess a large number of its members than if you assess a small number of members.

However, correctly characterizing a population does not mean that the results are important. For example, Flum and colleagues examined the records of 1,570,361 Medicare patients who underwent cholecystectomy during a 7-year period.[157] The investigators compared those patients who underwent an intraoperative cholangiography (IOC) to those who did not. (Performance of IOC is thought to increase the risk of common bile duct injury.) There were many statistically significant differences between patients who underwent IOC and those who did not (Table 9.3).

In fact, of the 12 comparisons shown in Table 9.3, nine are statistically significant at the $P < 0.001$ level and two are statistically significant at the $P \leq 0.05$. But are these differences important? No, most seem trivial. For example, 96.8%

---

[156] Shumaker, S.A., Legault, C., Rapp, S.R., et al. Estrogen plus progestin and the incidence of dementia and mild cognitive impairment in postmenopausal women. *J. Am. Med. Assoc.* 2003; 289: 2651–62.

[157] Flum, D.R., Dellinger, E.P., Cheadle, A., Chan, L., Koepsell, T. Intraoperative cholangiography and risk of common bile duct injury during cholecystectomy. *J. Am. Med. Assoc.* 2003; 289: 1639–44.

Table 9.3. Characteristics of patients with and without intraoperative cholangiography (IOC)

Variables	With IOC ($N = 613{,}706$)	Without IOC ($N = 956{,}655$)	P-value
Patient-level variables			
Age, mean (SD), (years)	71.7 (10.3)	71.2 (10.7)	0.001
Sex, (% of female)	62.6	63.2	0.001
Race, (% of white/non-Hispanic)	88.9	88.8	0.05
Complex biliary tract disease, (%)	10.9	11.0	0.05
Comorbidity index, mean (SD)	0.04 (0.22)	0.08 (0.24)	0.001
Surgeon-level variables			
Age, mean (SD), (years)	48.1 (9.3)	48.6 (9.6)	0.001
Sex, (% of male)	96.8	96.7	0.001
Percent performed in the surgeon's first 20 cholecystectomies	24.6	25.0	0.001
Case order, mean # (SD)	70.5 (61.3)	66.6 (57.7)	<0.001
General surgeon/surgical specialist	95.6	95.6	1.0
Surgeon board certified, (%)	82.6	79.6	<0.001
Years since surgeon graduated from medical school, mean (SD), (years)	21.8 (9.6)	22.3 (9.6)	<0.001

Data from Flum, D.R., et al. Intraoperative cholangiography and risk of common bile duct injury during cholecystectomy. *J. Am. Med. Assoc.* 2003; 289: 1639–44.

of patients who underwent IOC had a male surgeon versus 96.7% of patients who did not have an IOC. Although the difference is a trivial 0.1%, the difference is statistically significant at the $P < 0.001$ level. What is driving the statistical significance is the large sample size. Almost any difference no matter how trivial will be statistically significant if you have 1.5 million subjects!

Besides large sample sizes, very sensitive measures can lead to statistically significant, but clinically unimportant results. For example, a study of Alzheimer's disease found that patients given the medicine tacrine had statistically significant improvements on a scale very sensitive to cognitive changes (the cognitive scale of the Alzheimer's Disease Assessment) compared to patients who were given placebo. However, tacrine was not associated with improvements using more global measures of function such as the MiniMental State Examination.[158] Due to its very limited benefit, tacrine is not widely prescribed for patients with Alzheimer's disease.

---

[158] Qizilbash, N., Birks, J., Lopez Arrieta, J., Lewington S., Szeto, S. Tacrine for Alzheimer's disease (Cochrane Review). In: *The Cochrane Library* (Issue 3). 2003, Oxford: Update Software.

Tip

Make sure your effect size is clinically important before undertaking your study.

The best way to avoid a situation of having a statistically significant, but clinically unimportant result is to set an effect size *a priori* that is clinically important. Although this sounds obvious, much more attention is paid in both study design and study interpretation to the issue of statistical significance than to clinical significance.[159]

9.3 Can the results be statistically insignificant and clinically important?

Also: absolutely! There is nothing sacred about the conventionally used P-value of ≤ 0.05. There is no reason be dramatically more confident of a result that is significant at a P-value of 0.05 than a P-value of 0.06.

One way to avoid judging results based on a single threshold is to focus on the confidence intervals rather than the significance levels. The confidence intervals give you a sense of the range of results compatible with your data (Section 4.3). However, some people make the same mistake with confidence intervals as with P-values. That is, they dismiss any effect where the 95% CI don't exclude 1.0.

On the other hand, there does need to be some widely accepted threshold for deciding when chance is an unlikely explanation for a result. Otherwise, investigators would be tempted to move that threshold around, after the fact, to call their results statistically significant.

Tip

When clinically important differences do not reach statistical significance report the finding, but indicate that the difference did not reach statistical significance.

When you have a clinically important difference that does not reach statistical significance but is close to the conventional cut-off (e.g., $P = 0.07$ or the 95% CI includes one but excludes 0.98) report the finding, but indicate to the reader that it did not reach statistical significance.

For example, Kadish and colleagues tested the ability of an implantable cardioverter-defibrillator (ICD) to prevent deaths among patients with severe heart disease.[160] They randomized 458 patients with non-ischemic dilated cardiomyopathy, left ventricular dysfunction, and evidence of arrhythmias to receive standard medical therapy alone versus standard medical therapy plus a single-chamber ICD. Using proportional hazards regression, they found that the ICD group was less likely to die (relative hazard = 0.65). However, the 95% CI included 1 (0.40–1.06) and the P-value was 0.08.

Does this mean that ICDs do not save lives? No. What it does mean is that the study was underpowered for this outcome. When the investigators calculated their sample size they assumed that more than 50% of the deaths in the standard-therapy group would occur due to an arrhythmia. However, in the

[159] Man-Son-Hing, M., Laupacis, A., O'Rourke, K., et al. Determination of the clinical importance of study results. *J. Gen. Int. Med.* 2002; 17: 469–76.

[160] Kadish, A., Dyer, A., Daubert, J.P., et al. Prophylactic defibrillator implantation in patients with non-ischemic dilated cardiomyopathy. *New Engl. J. Med.* 2004; 350: 2151–8.

study, only a third of the deaths in the standard-therapy group were due to an arrhythmia. When the investigators used a more specific marker (Section 7.12) of the efficacy of ICD (sudden death due to an arrhythmia) they found a statistically significant decrease in deaths due to arrhythmias among the ICD recipients (relative hazard − 0.20; 95% CI = 0.06–0.71; $P = 0.006$).

On the other hand, some investigators mistakenly assert that their non-significant findings should be accepted as truth because if the sample size had been bigger, the P-value would have been statistically significant and the confidence intervals would have excluded 1.0. Although it is true that for a given effect size, a larger sample size will result in a smaller P-value (tossed coin example, Section 1.1) and narrow the confidence intervals, statistical significance testing takes into account the degree of uncertainty in the effect size at a given sample size. A larger sample size will result in less uncertainty but may also result in a different point estimate.

Special topics

10.1 What is the difference between the relative risk and the absolute risk?

> Absolute risk is more helpful in clinical situations than relative risk.

Relative risks (risk ratios and rate ratios (RR)) identify the risk factors for particular outcomes. However, they cannot tell you how likely an outcome is to occur, only how much more likely the outcome is to occur in one group than the other. Therefore, knowing the relative risk is not very helpful in clinical situations. In contrast, an absolute risk tells you how likely an outcome is to occur.

The difference between the relative risk and absolute risk is particularly great with rare diseases because a person at high relative risk of developing a disease (compared to an unexposed person) may still be very unlikely to develop that disease. For example, the relative risk of developing esophageal cancer is 40–125 higher among persons with Barrett esophagus. For persons newly diagnosed with Barrett esophagus this must sound like a certainty that they will develop cancer. In fact, the absolute risk of developing cancer if you have Barrett esophagus has been estimated at 0.5% per year (one in two hundred).[161] Despite the high relative risk, the absolute risk is low because esophageal cancer is a rare disease.

10.2 What other effect measures are available in addition to relative risk and absolute risk?

In addition to relative risk and absolute risk, several related effect measures are available. Each one characterizes the association between a risk factor and an outcome differently. The different measures, along with their meaning, and their uses, are shown in Table 10.1.

---

[161] Shaheen, N., Ransohoff, D.F. Gastroesophageal reflux, Barrett esophagus, and esophageal cancer. *J. Am. Med. Assoc.* 2002; 287: 1972–81.

Table 10.1. Comparison of different measures of effect

Effect measure	Meaning	Use
Absolute risk difference (attributable risk)	Incidence of disease that can be attributed to a particular exposure	Understand differences in risk due to differences in exposures
Attributable fraction	Proportion of disease due to a particular exposure	Understand importance of a particular factor on disease occurrence
Population attributable fraction	Incidence of disease due to a particular exposure in a community	Helpful in targeting public health interventions
Number needed to treat	Number of persons needed to be treated to prevent one outcome	Helpful in deciding whether it is worth adopting a clinical intervention

10.2.A Absolute risk difference

The absolute risk difference is the difference in the incidence between two groups:

$$
\begin{array}{c} \text{absolute risk} \\ \text{difference} \end{array} = \left(\begin{array}{c} \text{incidence among} \\ \text{exposed} \end{array} \right) - \left(\begin{array}{c} \text{incidence among} \\ \text{unexposed} \end{array} \right)
$$

> **Definition**
>
> Attributable risk tells you how much of the incidence of a disease can be attributed to a particular exposure.

Assuming that there is a causal relationship between the exposure and the outcome, the absolute risk difference tells you how much of the incidence of the disease is due to (can be attributed to) the exposure. For this reason it is also referred to as the attributable risk or the attributable risk in exposed persons.

In Section 5.9.A I reviewed a study comparing the risk of community-acquired pneumonia among patients exposed to acid suppressing drugs compared to persons not exposed. The investigators found that the incidence of pneumonia in patients exposed to acid suppressing drugs was 2.45 per 100 person years ($185/7562 \times 100$) and the incidence of pneumonia in unexposed patients was 0.55 per 100 person years ($5366/970,331 \times 100$). Therefore, the attributable risk (attributable to acid suppression medication) is 1.9 cases ($2.45 - 0.55$) per 100 person years.

10.2.B Attributable fraction (attributable risk percentage)

The attributable fraction (also known as the attributable risk percentage) tells us the proportion of a disease that is due to a particular exposure, assuming that the exposure causes the disease.[162] It is calculated as:

$$\frac{\text{attributable}}{\text{fraction}} = \frac{\text{incidence among exposed} - \text{incidence among unexposed}}{\text{incidence among exposed}}$$

Incidence in the formula can be incidence rate or incidence proportion.

Continuing with the example of acid suppressing drugs and pneumonia, the attributable fraction would be:

$$\frac{2.45 - 0.55}{2.45} = 0.78$$

In other words, 78% of the pneumonias that developed among the patients in the study can be attributed to acid suppressing drugs. This may seem very high to you because you are thinking that the attributable fractions for all the causes of pneumonia should add up to 100%. This is incorrect. The attributable fractions can exceed 100% because multiple causes can interact and result in disease (e.g., acid suppressing drugs in the setting of exposure to pneumococcus can cause pneumonia).[163]

This attributable fraction can also be stated in terms of RR, specifically:

$$\text{attributable fraction} = \frac{\text{RR} - 1.0}{\text{RR}}$$

To prove that the two ways of stating the attributable fraction are equivalent calculate the attributable fraction in terms of the RR. In Section 5.9.A we had calculated that the RR associated with exposure to acid suppressing drugs was 4.5. Therefore, he unadjusted attributable fraction would be:

$$\frac{4.5 - 1.0}{4.5} = 0.78$$

One advantage to the formula calculating attributable risk from the risk ratio is that the formula can be generalized so that you can approximate the attributable fraction from the odds ratio when it can be considered an approximation of the risk ratio (Section 5.2).

---

[162] Some authors define the attributable risk in the way I have defined the attributable fraction. It is best not to get distracted by the confusing nomenclature, and instead focus on the meaning of the comparison you are making.

[163] In fact, the sum of the attributable fractions is bounded by infinity. For more on this somewhat counter-intuitive idea see Rothman, K.J., Greenland, S. *Modern Epidemiology* (2nd edition). Philadelphia: Lippincott, Williams & Wilkins, 1998, pp. 12–14.

$$\text{attributable fraction}^* = \frac{OR - 1.0}{OR}$$
$$^*\text{Assuming outcome is uncommon } (<10\text{--}15\%)$$

This is very useful when you have performed logistic regression and have an odds ratio rather than a relative risk for a given exposure.

10.2.C Population attributable fraction

Population attributable fraction tells us the proportion of a disease that is due to a particular exposure in a population, assuming that the exposure causes the disease. This metric incorporates the prevalence of the risk factor such that interventions that decrease common risk factors reduce disease more than interventions that eliminate uncommon risk factors. Stated in a different way: if you had two interventions that halved the incidence of a particular disease, the intervention that decreased the more common risk factor would have a more powerful effect in the community than the intervention that eliminated the less common risk factor. The formula for population attributable fraction[164] is:

$$\frac{\text{population}}{\text{attributable fraction}} = \frac{\text{incidence in population} - \text{incidence in unexposed}}{\text{incidence in population}}$$

As with attributable fraction, incidence can be based on incidence rates or incidence proportions. The above formula can be rewritten mathematically[165] to more easily see the impact of the prevalence of the risk factor on the population attributable fraction:

$$\frac{\text{population}}{\text{attributable fraction}} = \frac{(\text{prevalence of risk factor in the population}) \times (RR - 1)}{[(\text{prevalence of risk factor in the population}) \times (RR - 1) + 1]}$$

The differences between risk ratios, attributable fraction, and population attributable fraction are illustrated by a population-based study of risk factors for uncontrolled hypertension (Table 10.2).[166] You can see that based on the relative risks, having no medical care is a stronger predictor of uncontrolled hypertension than being male. However, because only 10% of the sample had

---

[164] For more on attributable risk and population attributable risk see Kelsey, J.L., Whittemore, A.S., Evans, A.S., Douglas Thompson, W. *Methods in Observational Epidemiology* (2nd edition). Oxford: Oxford University Press, 1996, pp. 37–40.

[165] To see how: Szklo, M., Nieto, F.J. *Epidemiology: Beyond the Basics.* Gaithersburg, Maryland: Aspen Publication, pp. 101–5.

[166] Hyman, D.J., Pavlik, V.N. Characteristics of patients with uncontrolled hypertension in the United States. *New Engl. J. Med.* 2001; 345: 479–86.

Table 10.2. Risk factors for uncontrolled hypertension: comparison of relative risk and population attributable risk

	RR	Attributable fraction	Prevalence of risk factor	Population attributable fraction
Age ⩾65 years (versus <65 year)	2.08	0.52	0.44	0.32
Male sex (versus female sex)	1.30	0.23	0.43	0.12
No visits to physician in past 12 months (versus ⩾1 visits)	1.89	0.47	0.10	0.08

Data from Hyman, D.J., Pavlike, V.N. Characteristics of patients with uncontrolled hypertension in the United States. *New Engl. J. Med.* 2001; 345: 479–86.

no physician visits, compared to 43% of the sample being male, the population attributable fraction of having no physician visits was smaller than the effect of being male on explaining uncontrolled hypertension in the population. Therefore, improving access to physicians would have less of an impact on uncontrolled hypertension than sex.

10.2.D Number needed to treat

Number needed to treat is the number of persons who need to be treated over a given period of time to prevent one outcome (such as one stroke or one myocardial infarction).

The number needed to treat is calculated as:

$$\text{number needed to treat} = \frac{1}{\text{absolute risk difference}^*}$$

*See Section 10.2.A for calculation of absolute risk difference

> **Definition**
>
> Number needed to treat is the number of persons who need to be treated over a given period of time to prevent one outcome.

When it turns out that you have to treat thousands of people to prevent one bad outcome, you may decide that it is not worth the side effects, the cost, or the trouble to those who would have to take the medications. Conversely, when few have to be treated to confer a benefit, treatment is more attractive.

Often the same treatment will have substantially different numbers needed to treat depending on the likelihood that the patient will develop the disease. For example, Kumana et al. assessed the number needed to treat with statins to prevent coronary disease in different risk groups.[167] They found that the number

---

[167] Kumana, C.R., Cheung, B.M.Y., Lauder, I.J. Gauging the impact of statins using number needed to treat. *J. Am. Med. Assoc.* 1999; 282: 1899–901. The two primary sources of data for this article are: Scandinavian Simvastatin Survival Study Group. Randomized trial of cholesterol lowing in 4444 patients with coronary heart disease. *Lancet* 1994; 334: 1383–9; Owens, J.R., Clearfield, M., Weis, S. et al. Primary prevention of acute coronary events with lovastatin in men and women with average cholesterol levels: results of AFCAPS/TexCAPS. *J. Am. Med. Assoc.* 1998; 279: 1615–28.

Table 10.3. Efficacy of statins in prevention of coronary artery disease

	Relative risk associated with use of statins	Number needed to treat
Coronary artery disease and elevated cholesterol (secondary prevention)	0.66	63
No coronary artery disease and normal cholesterol (primary prevention)	0.63	256

needed to treat with statins per year to prevent a coronary event was 63 for persons with coronary heart disease and elevated cholesterol (secondary prevention) but was 256 for persons without coronary disease or elevated cholesterol (primary prevention) (Table 10.3). This difference is not conveyed by the relative risk, as both studies showed a similar relative reduction in the occurrence of coronary events (Table 10.3).

The number needed to treat is sensitive to the length of time of the intervention. Longer durations of treatment with an effective intervention will result in lower numbers needed to treat to prevent an outcome. However, longer durations of treatment generally also result in greater side effects and cost.

10.3 Do I need to use statistical analysis if I have population data?

The methods we have reviewed thus far for determining the statistical significance (P-values) of the different statistics discussed in this book (e.g., chi-squared, t-tests, linear regression) are based on inference. We infer the characteristics of the population based on a sample. The P-values and the 95% confidence intervals give us a sense of how likely it is that what we have found in our sample reflects the truth in the population.

But what if you have the whole population (or virtually the whole population) rather than a sample of that population? Does it still make sense to use inferential statistics? The short answer is no, although many people do.

For example, my colleagues and I at the San Francisco Health Department have performed a number of studies using the AIDS registry. As AIDS is a reportable disease and because San Francisco has a very aggressive surveillance program for AIDS that includes reviewing records at hospitals, private physicians office, laboratories, and performing matches with the National Death Index, our AIDS registry is more than 97% complete. Therefore, when we compare median survival for different groups of patients (e.g., younger versus older patients, homeless versus stably housed) we do not need to report *P*-values or 95% confidence intervals because the differences cannot be due to sampling (no sampling is performed – we have virtually the entire population).

On the other hand, if we wish to make inferences about the population of AIDS cases in the USA from the experience of AIDS cases in San Francisco, it would make sense to report *P*-values and confidence intervals.

10.4 How do I choose what statistical program to use for analyzing data?

Any of the widely available commercial statistical programs (e.g., BMDP, S-Plus, SAS, SPSS, and STATA) perform all the analyses that most clinical researchers will need. Therefore, the major determinant of what package you will want to use will be whether you are working with an established research group or on your own.

If you are working with an established group, use the same package as the other members of your group so that you can ask your colleagues for help.

If you are starting out on your own, choose a package based on ease and cost. Based on these factors, Epi Info is hard to beat. As it was created by the Centers for Disease Control and Prevention (CDC) for field investigations of disease outbreaks, it takes you smoothly from the stage of writing a questionnaire to entering the data and analyzing it. It is free and can be downloaded from the Internet (www.cdc.gov/epiinfo/).

However, Epi Info has limitations. If your data are already entered into a spreadsheet it can be hard to use. It does not perform sophisticated analyses such as proportional hazards regression, Poisson regression, or generalized estimation equations. Even for simpler analyses, it has a more limited repertoire of analyses (e.g., it does not perform McNemar's test). Nonetheless, you can always enter your data with Epi Info, perform preliminary analyses, and then export the data to another statistical program to perform more specialized analyses.

A more comprehensive data package that is also available free is R (http://www.r-project.org/). It is modeled after S-Plus and, like S-Plus, provides excellent graphing capability. It will take you longer to learn R, but it does a much more extensive array of analyses than Epi Info. If you have data drawn from a stratified, clustered, or multistage sample design (Section 5.10), the statistical program SUDAAN is particularly useful.

At times you may have bivariate data in summary form for which you need to compute a statistic. There are several programs on the web that can perform chi-squared and Fisher's exact from a cross-tabulation table, or a McNemer's test from the tabulated number of discordant pairs.[168]

---

[168] See, for example: Simple Interactive Statistical Analysis at http://home.clar.net/sisa/sampshlp.htm

Publishing research

11.1 How do I write my study up for publication?

Having completed a well-designed, well-analysed study you are now ready to write your results up for publication. This is a critical step: your research cannot improve clinical care unless it is read and understood.

Several excellent guides on how to write up your results already exist.[169] I offer only the following pointers:

1. The easiest way to write a first draft of a research paper is to find two or three studies similar to yours that have been published in the same journal (or other media format) that you intend to submit your paper to. Choose papers that use a similar study design as yours (i.e., if you are writing up the results of an observational cohort choose a paper that also uses an observational cohort design). It is also helpful, but not essential, for the papers to be on the same topic as yours.

   Now, before writing each section of the paper (e.g., Introduction, Methods) read the same section in each of the three examples. Next write your section mimicking the style of the three papers you have read. Remember that creativity is a very desirable quality when writing novels, but not when writing up the results of clinical research. When I want creative writing, I read Virginia Wolff. When I read a journal I want the information to be in a format that I can absorb efficiently. Remember that imitating the style and format of another paper is not plagiarism – plagiarism is copying another person's words or ideas.

2. Write the first draft of your article, using the technique above, *prior* to collecting your data! This is the best way to make sure that you have not omitted any crucial variables from your data collection and that you have anticipated

---

[169] My favorite is: Browner, W.S. *Publishing and Presenting Clinical Research*. Philadelphia: Lippincott, Williams & Wilkins: 1999. My advice is similar to his (he was my mentor) but he provides more extensive guidance. For excellent tips on manuscript submission: Samet, J.M. Dear Author – advice from a retiring editor. *Am. J. Epidemiol.* 1999; 150: 433–6. Specifications on how to submit your paper will usually be available at the journal's web site; a compendium of journal requirements for submission is available at www.mco.edu/lib/instr/libinsta.html. Also many journals follow the same format: Uniform Requirements for Manuscripts Submitted to Biomedical Journals available at www.icmje.org.

the limitations of your study at a time when you still may be able to fix these problems. It will also help make your data analysis more efficient by focusing you on those analyses key to your manuscript.

Obviously, if you write your paper prior to collecting your data, it will have some large holes in it. But you certainly do not need the data to write the introduction (the introduction frames your question) or to write the Methods section (this section describes how you have enrolled subjects, collected data, etc.).

Draft the Results section by stating the analyses that you intend to do. For example: Bivariate analyses showed that marathon runners (were/were not) younger and less likely to smoke than couch potatoes. In a logistic regression analysis, adjusting for age, weight, blood pressure, cholesterol level, smoking status, marathon runners (were/were not) less likely to develop coronary artery disease than couch potatoes.

For your discussion, focus on the limitations of your analysis. For example, a limitation of our study was that sexual behaviors were based on self-report. However, to minimize bias due to clients answering in a way designed to please the interviewers (social-desirability bias) we had clients answer questions about their sexual behaviors using a computer entry system (Section 3.3).

3. Shorter is better when it comes to the Introduction and the Conclusion. Not so for the Methods. Reviewers and other experts in your field are likely to judge your work by the Methods sections. (In contrast, casual journal readers will skip the Methods section.) Take pains to describe your study fully in the Methods.

4. Do not repeat the same information in the text and the tables. If you can adequately describe the result in the text without having your manuscript read like a financial report, do so. If a table is required to show your data, state only the major trends in the Results section.

5. Admit to all pertinent biases in the Discussion section. Reviewers and editors will be more forgiving of biases that you recognize than those that you ignore. Also, identifying each bias gives you the opportunity to defend your study. Explain to your reader, if possible, why the bias would not be expected to have a substantial effect on your analyses. For example: We do not believe that our results could be due to differential loss of subjects between the treatment and the non-treatment group because the percentage and characteristics of subjects lost to follow-up in the two groups was similar. If your best defense is not very convincing then acknowledge the bias and omit the defense. Some biases cannot be defended.

6. If your observational study identifies a potentially causal association, then the major limitation of your study is that the statistical association is due to

something other than cause–effect. Discuss each of the threats to causality (e.g., confounding, reverse causality) listed in Section 9.1 and cite additional data, if possible, to defend why you do not believe that this threat is operating in your study. For example, if there is a significant time lag between the measurement of the risk factor and the development of the disease, it is unlikely that the disease caused the risk factor or that you failed to exclude persons who already had the disease at the start of the study.

7. Once you have a first draft that you are happy with, circulate it to your co-authors. Ask them to read it and comment. Incorporate their comments into a final draft. Do not be surprised if your co-authors disagree as to what changes to make. Do your best to talk out the issues to reach consensus. The process itself sometimes results in a better resolution than anyone had initially proposed. Ultimately, it is the first author who usually makes the final decision when opinions among the authors conflict. This is also a good time to ask a biostatistician to review the paper, especially the methods and the results, to be certain that you have performed and reported your analysis correctly.

8. Before sending your paper to a journal, ask at least two colleagues who have not been involved in the project to review it. Ask them to be as critical as they would be if they were reviewing it for a journal (this is important because it is often difficult to be critical of your friends). Honest criticism is what you want before submitting a manuscript. It gives you the opportunity to improve your work before it is judged by reviewers who will surely be more critical than your friends. Some research groups organize an internal peer review process in a seminar format. This is a very good way of getting objective feedback. If it is available to you, use it!

11.2 How do I determine authorship for the paper?

Authorship should be based on intellectual effort. Although there is no one standard on the amount of effort that constitutes authorship, the International Committee of Medical Journal Editors recommends that all authors should:

1. have made substantial contributions to conception and design, or acquisition of data, or analysis, and interpretation of data;

2. have written the article or revised it critically for important intellectual content;

3. have approved the final version of the paper.

To avoid "vanity" authorships many journals require that all authors certify that they have fulfilled these three criteria. A person whose sole contribution is acquisition of funding, data collection, or supervision of personnel should not be included as an author, but should be named in the Acknowledgement section.

Among the authors, the first author should be the person who put in the most intellectual effort, the second author the second most effort, etc. Usually the first author writes the manuscript and takes responsibility for corresponding with the journal editors prior to publication as well as answering questions about the work from other scientists, the media, and members of the public.

Often the epidemiologist or statistician who conducts the analysis is the second author and the most senior person in the research group is the last author. However, this is by no means a uniform rule and it is best for the order of authorship to reflect the level of effort of each author.

11.3 How do I resolve disagreements about authorship?

There is an old joke about academia that I find instructive. Why is there so much infighting among academics? Because the stakes are so small!

The most difficult conflicts are usually about who will be the first author. The reason is that the order of authorship is not an interval scale! The perceived difference between first author and second author is much greater than that between the second and third author, third and fourth author, etc.

> **Tip**
>
> Decide authorship at the beginning of a project.

The best way to avoid conflicts about authorship is to decide on authorship at the start of a project. That way everyone can agree on what their responsibilities on the project will be and on how those contributions will be recognized. If a particular investigator does not agree, he or she may decline to participate.

Although this rule is simple and sound, it does not always work. Investigators leave and new ones join the team. Someone planning initially to direct a project cannot do so due to other demands. A portion of the project turns out to be more time consuming than expected. An unplanned analysis turns out to be more compelling than the original question. With any of these scenarios you may be left with two or more authors who feel they should be first author.

The first step with such a disagreement is for the two investigators to meet together with or without the other members of the research team to discuss openly why each feels they should be the first author. If the project is likely to produce more than one publication, perhaps it is possible for each to be first author on one paper.

If they cannot agree, they should ask one or two colleagues to help them mediate the decision. Ideally these should be senior investigators with lots of publication experience and no involvement in the project. The two authors should agree to abide by the decision of the mediator(s). Each author should present to the mediator the reason that he or she should be first author. The mediator should ask clarifying questions about the involvement each had in the project and make a final decision.

What should never happen (but does) is that an authorship conflict slows or prevents the publication of the work. This is a tremendous disservice to the subjects and to science, and selfishly places the needs of the investigators above both.

You may also have a disagreement with someone who feels that they should be included in a manuscript but you do not agree. This can be especially difficult if the person who wishes to be included is the head of your research group (i.e., the one who will determine your salary, where your office is located, whether you will be promoted, etc.).

The "right" answer is that if you are the first author and that person has not contributed in a substantial way to the manuscript, you should not include them. You might be able to pre-empt a request to be included as an author by asking the person's permission to acknowledge his or her contribution at the end of the paper.

When this doesn't satisfy the would-be author, giving him or her the statement required by most journals to be signed by all authors verifying that they have made a substantial intellectual contribution to the work may result in he or she bowing out gracefully. Sadly, this is not always the case. If the person is willing to sign that they contributed in a substantial way, it is difficult for a junior author to be the one to say no. In difficult circumstances such as this, you should either allow them to be included (and promise yourself you will never seek vanity authorship when you are the head of the research team) or seek advice from a senior colleague in a different research group on how to proceed.

There may also be disagreements about the order of authors after the first author. This type of disagreement is generally less rancorous because exact order does not have the same importance as being the first author or the significance of being included/excluded as an author. The issue can usually be resolved through open discussion and comparisons of contributions.

11.4 How do I decide what journal to send the paper to?

The short answer is: send it to the best journal that your paper stands a reasonable chance of getting accepted to. I will spend the rest of this section trying to help you figure out what constitutes "best."

Factors to consider in deciding which journal to send your paper to include:
- Prestige of journal
- Reaching your target audience
- Publication time
- Availability of journal.

11.4.A Prestige of journal

I have listed prestige first, not because I think it is the most important, but because it is generally the first thing academic researchers consider. For better or for worse, the university system of promotion and tenure tends to reward those who publish their research in the most prestigious journals. And to the extent that it is more difficult to publish research in the most prestigious journals, it is an *imperfect* measure of the quality of your work. It is imperfect because other factors besides the quality of your work will influence whether your work gets accepted. Who you are, who you know, how topical your work is, whether it is the kind of work that the journal editor is interested in, as well as luck, will all affect whether you get an acceptance or a rejection letter. Although the prestige of a journal is subjective, your senior colleagues will have no trouble specifying the most prestigious journals in your field.

11.4.B Reaching target audience

Reaching your target audience is, in my opinion, the most important factor in choosing a journal. If you are trying to influence the practice of pulmonologists, you need to publish in a journal read by pulmonologists (e.g., *American Review of Respiratory Diseases*). If you are trying to reach policy makers you need to publish your work in a journal read by them (e.g., *Health Affairs*). Closely matching your article to the readership of the journal will also increase the chance that the journal will accept your article.

Publishing in a journal with a large circulation (e.g., *New England Journal of Medicine, Journal of American Medical Association (JAMA)*) is one way to increase the impact of your work. It will alert persons to your findings who do not read specialty journals. However, journals with large circulations look for articles of general interest and may reject a paper on a topic of narrow interest even if the work is impeccable.

11.4.C Speed of publication

Three major factors affect the time from the submission of a manuscript to its publication:
1. the speed of the journal in reviewing manuscripts;
2. the time between acceptance and publication;
3. the number of different journals you submit your paper to prior to it being accepted for publication.

Some journals respond more rapidly than others to submitted manuscripts. Journals with strong editorial review will often respond quickly (in the negative!)

without even sending the paper out to review. Although this may sound harsh, it is actually a gift. It is much better to have an article rejected after a month than after 6 months. Some journals also require that their reviewers be disciplined and respond back in a reasonable period of time.

Some journals have a backlog of accepted articles. Other journals go to press infrequently. Such journals are unable to publish work quickly even when the review process goes smoothly. Although the review process is unpredictable, almost all journals should be able to tell you about how long it will take for an accepted article to be published.

Rapid publication is especially important when you have a novel finding with major clinical applications. To guarantee the rapid publication of findings that are likely to change practice, some journals have a specific fast track. The fast track generally has a higher threshold for publication to discourage everyone from submitting his or her work under the fast track.

Often the greatest determinant of how rapidly a piece of research is published is how many journals you must submit it to before it is accepted. When you have time critical work, do not send it to multiple journals where it may have a relatively low chance of success.

On the other hand, for some articles the exact time of publication is not so crucial. With such studies you can afford to take a chance and submit it to a journal or journals where it may not have a high probability of getting accepted.

11.4.D Availability of journal

The web has caused a major shift in how people think about the availability of a journal. It used to be that the circulation of a journal was of crucial significance in choosing where to submit a manuscript because if it were published in a journal with a small circulation, few would read it and it would have little impact on the field. Now as long as the journal is indexed by Index Medicus (or one of the analogous databases in other fields such as the Social Sciences Citation Index) the abstract will be available online at a site such as PubMed or SOCIAL SCISEARCH. Some abstracts include the e-mail address of the author, allowing the reader to e-mail you to obtain a copy of your work.

One way to increase access to your work is to publish it in a journal that provides free internet access to the full article. Several journals (*Lancet, British Medical Journal*) allow all their contents to be reviewed free on-line. Also there are an increasing number of internet open access journals (http://www. biomedcentral.com/) that in addition to publishing articles more rapidly (articles are usually posted immediately following journal acceptance) offer the advantage that anyone can download the full version of the paper for free.

Internet access is especially important if your study has relevance to researchers and clinicians in underdeveloped countries, where access to journals through medical libraries is limited.

11.5 What if my paper is rejected but I am asked to revise and resubmit it?

Be happy! It is rare that any of us have our work accepted on the first submission. Although a revise and resubmit letter is no guarantee of publication, it is the first step to having your paper accepted.

The key to getting your paper over this last hurdle is to adequately address the comments of the editors and the reviewers. In doing this, try not to be defensive. Pretend you are a salesperson: assume the customer (in this case the editor or the reviewer) is right. In other words, do not focus on proving that you were right. For example, if a reviewer complains that no information about recruitment was included in the manuscript, but you know it was included, do not rail against the lazy reviewer. Assume that you did not do a very good job of explaining it. Review that section and see if there is a way you can explain the issue more clearly.

Of course, if the suggestion of the reviewer or the editor is wrong, then you need to explain why you have not chosen to make the change.

In your response to the editor, begin by thanking him or her for inviting you to resubmit your paper and for the suggestions of how to improve the paper. Address each point raised by the editor and the reviewers using numbers so as to make it easy for the editor to follow the changes. With each comment, first explain what the reviewer/editor has asked you to do, then explain how you addressed the issue, and finally include the actual section of the manuscript that you changed (with the page number) so that the editor can review the changes you have made without having to search through the revised manuscript. For example:

Dear Editor:

Thank you for inviting us to resubmit our manuscript: "The impact of designated bicycle lanes on frequency of bicycling to work". We appreciate your detailed review of the manuscript.

Below we explain each of the issues raised by the reviewers and how we have incorporated their suggestions into their manuscript.

1. Reviewer "A" is concerned that the increases in bicycling to work that we found may not be due to the creation of the designated bicycle lanes but may instead be due to a greater societal interest in fitness.

To address this concern we compared the number of times people bicycled in the park pre- and post-creation of the bicycle lanes and found no difference.

We have added the following to the Results section:

There were no differences in the frequency that persons stated that they bicycled in the park pre- and post-creation of the designated bicycle paths (median = 1.3 times per month versus 1.2 times per month, respectively; $P > 0.20$) (p. 13).

We have added to the Discussion section:

Although there was a substantial difference in the frequency of bicycling to work with the creation of the designated bicycle paths, we found no difference in frequency of bicycling in the park. If the increases we saw in bicycling to work were due to a general societal interest in fitness, we would have expected to also find an increase in bicycling in the park (p. 15).

11.6 What if my paper is rejected?

Any rejection, professional or personal, is painful. Rejection of a manuscript can be particularly difficult because of the years of effort that go into planning, conducting, and writing up the results of a study. Besides sadness, you may feel anger towards the editors or the reviewers for failing to appreciate the value of your work.

Although these feelings are natural, they are not particularly helpful in deciding your next step. For this reason, it is often best to put the rejection letter aside after reading it and return to it when your feelings have subsided a bit. (I would hasten to add that this is a good strategy in dealing with many of life's difficulties.)

Once some time has elapsed, reread the reviews and the manuscript. Try to determine as specifically as you can why your paper got rejected. Generally, the reason will fall into one of the following groups:

1. insufficient interest on the part of the journal,
2. an unfair review,
3. flaws in the paper that you can address,
4. flaws in the paper that you cannot address.

You will know that your paper got rejected due to insufficient interest on the part of the journal if the Editors did not send it out for review or if the reviews were positive but your article was still rejected. In this case, it is best to quickly resubmit your article to another journal, ideally one that is more focused on the topic of your manuscript.

Although researchers often feel that the reviews of their paper were unfair, in my experience, this is rarely the case. Harsh, critical, unforgiving: yes. Lazy, biased: sometimes. Unfair: rarely. Most top-notch journals send papers out to multiple reviewers; if all the reviewers have the same negative feeling about your article, there probably is a problem, if not with your findings, then with your ability to communicate your findings.

However, it is possible to have several positive reviews and one very negative one that you believe is unfair. If this is the case, you may try to appeal the decision of the Editor.

Top-notch journals must reject many more papers than they can accept. A paper that is at the borderline may fall to one side or the other depending on the mood of the editorial board at the time your article is being considered by them. If you decide to appeal a decision, it should be based on the importance of the work appearing in that journal. Sometimes it helps if the senior author writes the appeal letter explaining why he or she feels the work is important to publish. Remember, appealing a rejection should only be done if you received mostly positive reviews. Otherwise you are wasting your time and that of the editor. It should also be done in a very respectful way or you run the risk of developing a reputation for being difficult.

If your article was rejected due to flaws that you can address, fix them and resubmit to another journal. If it was rejected due to flaws that you cannot address, you need to decide your next step. Sometimes, a combination of admitting the flaws clearly in the Discussion section and submitting it to a less prominent journal will result in it being published. Sometimes markedly shortening the manuscript into a letter will result in publication. However, if your paper gets rejected multiple times (including as a letter) because of the same flaws, file the manuscript and get to work on a new project.

> **Tip**
>
> If your paper gets rejected multiple times because of the same flaws file the manuscript and get to work on a new project.

11.7 How should I deal with the media?

Many researchers are unnecessarily afraid of the press. They worry that their results will be misquoted or sensationalized. To avoid this possibility they hide from the media. This is a big mistake as media attention can amplify the impact of your work (not to mention providing unimaginable pleasure to your family and friends!). Also journalists, especially those who write on medicine and science topics, are genuinely interested in correctly capturing the findings of your study – after all, translation of science into lay terms is their job.

Some journals routinely provide advance copies of manuscripts along with press releases to the major media outlets. This makes your job somewhat easier. However, if your journal is not planning to publicize your article and you feel that your article has significance to lay persons, prepare a press release.

Generally, you will want to send out your press release before the date of publication of your article or the presentation of your data at a conference so that media outlets will have sufficient time to prepare their presentations in time for the release date. On the other hand, you may not want the media coverage to begin until the

> A press release should contain an explanation of the findings in lay terms and why they are important, a quote from the principal authors and/or others in the field, and information on who should be called for further questions (along with telephone and fax numbers, and e-mail address).

Your press release should include the embargo date (if any).

date of publication or presentation. This is especially true of important clinical findings. It is very disconcerting as a clinician when your patients ask you about the results of a trial they read about in the newspaper and you have no data source to use in evaluating the claims in the newspaper. To avoid this situation, the press release should state if the material is embargoed (cannot be released) until a particular date. Although, embargoes cannot be enforced, almost all professional media people will respect an embargoed report because they understand that without embargoes it would be impossible to brief the media ahead of the release of data.

Send your press packet to media outlets (television, radio, print, internet) in your area and nationally/internationally (if the findings warrant this). Follow-up the press release with calls to media people you think might be interested (e.g., the science writer at your local newspaper).

Most journalists will want to interview you on the results. Do not be frightened. They are not trying to catch you off guard. An interview gives you a chance to answer any questions, correct misinterpretations, and help the journalist shape the story.

You may find that a journalist will try to push you to generalize your findings beyond the scope of your work. Do not fall for it. If you are asked a question that goes beyond the data simple state: "the study did not address that question" or "I have no data on that question, but our data do show . . ."

Tip

Before your interview determine the three most important points of the paper.

Prior to doing an interview, determine the three most important points of the paper. Then make sure you state these three points during the interview. If you are asked a question that you are not comfortable answering, simply state one of the points.

After the press coverage has passed, call or write to those media people who covered your story well and thank them for doing so. Building a positive relationship with help you the next time you want to get coverage for a story.

Also, do not blame the print writers for the headlines in their newspaper. Someone else does these and they often do not fit the article.[170]

---

[170] For more detailed advice on working with the media see: Stamm, K., Williams, J.W., Noel, P.H., Rubin R. Helping journalists get it right: a physician's guide to improving health care reporting. *J. Gen. Intern. Med.* 2003; 18: 138–45.

Conclusion

12.1 Would you review the steps for designing and analyzing data from a clinical study?

Step 1   Choose a question that you are genuinely interested in knowing the answer to.

Step 2   Perform a literature search, review the published work, and speak to the experts in the field to learn of unpublished work.

Step 3   State your question in terms of a null and an alternative hypothesis.

Step 4   Choose a study design by considering the advantages and disadvantages of the different methods (Chapter 2).

Step 5   Determine the type of univariate, bivariate, and multivariable analyses you will need to perform (Chapters 4–6).

Step 6   Perform a sample size calculation (Chapter 7).

Step 7   Develop a study manual (Section 3.2).

Step 8   Submit your research protocol to an institutional review board for approval (Section 2.12).

Step 9   Develop data entry screens (Section 3.3).

Step 10   Collect your data (Section 3.2).

Step 11   Enter your data (Section 3.4).

Step 12   Clean, recode, and transform your data, and derive any variables you will need (Sections 3.5–3.8).

Step 13   Review the distribution of all of your variables (Section 4.1).

Step 14   Conduct univariate, then bivariate, and finally multivariate analyses (Chapters 4–6).

Step 15   Write up your results (Section 11.1).

Step 16   Send out for publication (Section 11.4).

Step 17   Revise and resubmit (Sections 11.5–11.6).

Step 18   Develop a media strategy to coincide with the publication of your paper (Section 11.7).

Step 19   Bask in your glory!

Index